HVAC SYSTEMS
MOLD
&
THE INDOOR ENVIRONMENT

A Comprehensive Guide to
Better Indoor Air Quality

Christopher Thome CIEC, CVI, VSMR

HVAC Systems, Mold & the Indoor Environment

A Comprehensive Guide to Better Indoor Air Quality

Copyright © 2025 by JenCar Enterprises

ISBN: 979-8-9920684-0-5

Disclaimer: This book is not intended to provide or replace medical advice. The information contained herein should not be used to diagnose, treat, prevent, or cure any disease or medical condition. Following the advice provided may not offer complete protection in all situations or against all health hazards associated with indoor air pollution. The mention of any trade names or commercial products does not imply endorsement or recommendation for use. These insights are just my opinions as a multi-state licensed air conditioning contractor, state licensed mold assessor, Council certified Indoor Environmental Consultant (CIEC), Certified Ventilation Inspector (CVI), and remediation professional. They are based on decades of investigation and successful projects resolving complex indoor air quality issues. Individual results may vary. An assessment by a qualified professional is always recommended.

Dedication

This book is dedicated to my wife, best friend, and business partner, Brandy Thome. Her inspiration and unwavering support made this journey possible. Thank you for motivating me to follow my passion and write about a subject I truly care about.

Acknowledgments

I would like to express my appreciation to the environmental assessors, remediators, and health care professionals who have put their trust in me to help their clients navigate HVAC-related indoor air quality challenges. Additionally, I am thankful to the many clients who have relied on me for assistance with their indoor air quality issues over the last 25 years. While I have chosen not to disclose specific names or businesses in this book, their trust and collaboration have been invaluable.

I'm also grateful to my dad, Robert Thome, for his calm guidance and continual support in all my endeavors.

Affiliations

- ACCA – Air Conditioning Contractors of America

- AHRI – Air-Conditioning, Heating and Refrigeration Institute

- ACGIH – American Conference of Governmental Industrial Hygienists

- ACAC – American Council for Accredited Certification

- AIHA – American Industrial Hygiene Association

- ALA – American Lung Association

- AMA – American Medical Association

- ANSI – American National Standards Institute

- ASHRAE – American Society of Heating, Refrigeration, and Air-Conditioning Engineers

- ASTM – American Society for Testing and Materials

- BOMA – Building Owners and Managers Association

- CSLB – The California Contractors State Licensing Board

- CDC – Centers for Disease Control and Prevention

- DBPR – Florida Department of Business and Professional Regulation

- EAA – Environmental Assessment Association

- EPA – Environmental Protection Agency

- FRACCA – Florida Refrigeration and Air Conditioning Contractors Association

- IAQA – Indoor Air Quality Association

- IICRC – Institute of Inspection, Cleaning and Restoration Certification

- ICC – International Code Council, Inc.

- ISEAI – International Society for Environmentally Acquired Illness

- NADCA – National Air Duct Cleaners Association

- NAFA – National Air Filtration Association

- NFPA – National Fire Protection Association

- NIH – National Institute of Health

- NIOSH – National Institute of Occupational Safety and Health

- NORMI – National Organization of Remediators and Mold Inspectors

- NYCDH – New York City Department of Health

- NAIMA – North American Insulation Manufacturers Association

- OSHA – Occupational Safety and Health Administration

- RACCA – Refrigeration and Air Conditioning Contractors Association

- SMACNA – Sheet Metal & Air Conditioning Contractors' National Association

- WHO – World Health Organization

Professional Experience

1990: Desert Storm Veteran, U.S. Army, 82nd Airborne Division

1999: BS in Psychology, The University of Tampa

1999: EPA 608 Universal Certification

2001: NADCA – Air Systems Cleaning Specialist, ASCS

2003: NADCA – Ventilation Systems Mold Remediator, VSMR

NADCA – Certified Ventilation Inspector, CVI

2004: IAQA – Certified Mold Remediator, CMR

2014: CA State Licensed Air Conditioning Contractor

2016: FL State Licensed Air Conditioning Contractor

2025: ACAC – Council-certified Indoor Environmental Consultant, CIEC

2025: FL State Licensed Mold Assessor

Christopher Thome is the Co-Founder and CEO of EnviroAir Systems, an HVAC mold inspection, remediation and indoor environmental consulting company.

Contents

Introduction

Mold, HEPA filters, air purifiers, UV lights and indoor air quality are topics that have become increasingly relevant today. Who doesn't want the air they breathe in their home or work to be clean and free of contaminants, or at least to have some control over them? But what does "good indoor air quality" really mean? How can you tell if your air conditioning system is delivering clean and comfortable air? If issues arise, who should you hire to diagnose the problem and outline a resolution? How can you ensure the work has been done correctly? And how do you know if the equipment, such as filters, air purifiers, or UV lights, is effectively improving your indoor air quality? If these questions have crossed your mind, you're in the right place. This book aims to provide clear, actionable answers in a straightforward roadmap. So, where do we begin?

The process for improving the indoor air quality begins with a thorough HVAC inspection and environmental impact assessment (EIA) of the heating, ventilation and air conditioning (HVAC) system and surrounding areas to identify any negative influences on the indoor environment or the HVAC system itself. This inspection will provide the information needed to make recommendations specific to each individual situation. This creates a clear path to achieving consistent, positive results and a successful outcome. Leaving health concerns related to indoor air quality to chance is a risky proposition. With nearly half my life spent investigating and resolving challenging indoor air quality issues, I'm here to help you achieve the indoor air quality you deserve.

This can be a stressful time digesting the information regarding your home's deficiencies, especially when these issues impact your health. Data-driven results can alleviate that stress, offering peace of mind that your environment is safe. With proper monitoring and routine maintenance of the HVAC system, achieving, controlling, and maintaining good indoor air quality becomes a manageable reality.

My Story

My name is Chris Thome, and I have been in the indoor air quality industry for over 25 years. After graduating from the University of Tampa, I began my career with an air conditioning company, an unexpected turn that nonetheless set me on the successful path I continue to follow today. My first decade in the indoor air quality industry was dedicated to evaluating and remediating HVAC systems for various facilities, including hospitals, schools, businesses, and industrial sites. I have successfully completed projects across a range of building classifications – residential, commercial, industrial, healthcare, educational, agricultural, and marine. After years of crawling through moldy ductwork, the excitement began to wane, and I was eager for new challenges.

During this period, I met my wife, and we moved to California's Central Valley, one of the most productive agricultural regions in the world; responsible for over half of the fruits, vegetables, and nuts grown in the United States. With around 250 crops cultivated across some 1,500 farms, I wondered how I could apply my indoor air quality expertise in this setting.

We started an environmental consulting business focused on providing indoor air quality solutions for early crop production indoor facilities. These environments demand precise air quality to ensure these starter plants are the healthiest and strongest they can be. This consulting work allowed me to refine my skills in maintaining these spaces free of mold and other contaminants detrimental to optimal plant growth.

These environments require a solid understanding of temperature, humidity, building pressurization, particulate control, carbon dioxide management, microbial control, and other factors essential for indoor hydroponic farming. Through effective temperature regulation, filtration, humidification, dehumidification, air purification, and strategic airflow management, I created perfect indoor environments. After several years in this demanding field, we decided to return to Florida to apply my expertise in a state heavily affected by mold.

Upon my return to Florida and after obtaining my Florida state air conditioning contractor's license; in 2016, we started EnviroAir Systems, a company dedicated to helping people with their HVAC systems and addressing their impact on the indoor environment and people's health. Our company quickly established itself as the leader in diagnosing and resolving indoor air quality problems related to HVAC systems facing high humidity and mold challenges.

Today, we work in conjunction with mold assessors, mold remediators, health care providers, and others, to address the challenges of contaminated environments. We offer a third-party clearance guarantee to ensure our work is done right, with verifiable results. For those grappling with microbial-related problems, lab results confirming the absence of mold or confirming acceptable ecological conditions within the HVAC system and environment can provide much-needed reassurance.

EnviroAir Systems' ongoing success has allowed me to share my comprehensive understanding of diagnosing and addressing challenging indoor air quality issues. We have assisted countless individuals suffering from Chronic Inflammation Response Syndrome (CIRS) and Lyme Disease, compromised immune systems, chemical and mold sensitivities, asthma, and other respiratory concerns related to the air they breathe at home and work.

What to Expect from This Book

This book is a roadmap to understanding the process involved in improving indoor air quality, with a focus on HVAC systems and their role in creating healthy, comfortable environments. You will learn about common indoor air quality challenges. Each chapter explores a key topic, from understanding the basics of indoor air quality like humidity, particulate control and HVAC components to what an overall remediation project may entail. Whether you're a homeowner, or business owner, this book provides guidance on navigating challenging health related concerns involving the HVAC system and your indoor environment.

By the end of this book, you will have clarity on how to achieve and maintain optimal indoor air quality, so you are empowered to make informed decisions and take effective action to improve the air you breathe.

Chapter 1

My Journey to Becoming an Indoor Air Quality "Professional"

My introduction to the indoor air quality field began in 1999 when I started working for an air conditioning company that also provided air duct cleaning services. On my first day of training, I was introduced to a tool that resembled a spinning mop, which was used to clean the ductwork. I watched the guy training me as he "upsold" the customer a sanitizing treatment after we moped out the ductwork. I thought to myself, "Sanitized ductwork? This must be some good stuff."

Once the AC fan was turned on, an atomizer or fogging machine was used to disperse the sanitizer into the air return, allowing it to travel throughout the system and into the home. As the fog filled the space so thickly that it became hard to breathe, everyone in the house dashed for the door, eager to escape outside.

Within a week, I found myself out on my own, tasked with cleaning, sanitizing, repairing, and replacing ductwork and air conditioning equipment. I did my best with minimal guidance, operating in a learn-as-you-go environment. There were no formal training programs, standards, or protocols to follow. I began to think, "If I had my own equipment, I could provide a better service." So, just a month or two into the job, I made the decision to give my two-week notice.

After leaving my first HVAC job, I went into debt by purchasing an air duct cleaning machine and began cleaning ductwork. At the time, I didn't hold an air conditioning contractor's license, which is required by most states for this type of work. Florida mandates a state license, so I partnered with a successful company that was looking to expand. I operated in the northern region of the state, adhering to the National Air Duct Cleaners Association (NADCA) standards.

Established in 1989 and now comprised of more than 1,500 member companies, NADCA is dedicated to establishing protocols and procedures and providing guidance and minimum standards for the assessment, cleaning, and restoration of HVAC systems. The cleaning process I employed is known as source contamination removal, as detailed in the current NADCA Standard ACR2025, an international standard used all over the world.

At that time, most of my projects were classified as commercial. I worked in hospitals, including NICU wards and operating room wings, schools during summer breaks, and industrial facilities with air handlers large enough to park several vans inside. I also consulted on the ventilation ductwork for a Navy ship, a Coast Guard vessel, and several private yachts. Over the years, I've been involved in numerous projects, including work for financial institutions and banks, religious churches and temples, upscale white tablecloth restaurants, military and government facilities, agricultural farms, countless residential homes and even an extremely challenging restoration project for a company that grows crystals for NASA.

During my initial years in this industry, I earned the Air Systems Cleaning Specialists (ASCS) certification through NADCA. Soon after, in 2003, NADCA introduced the Ventilation Systems Mold Remediator (VSMR) and the Certified Ventilation Inspector (CVI) certifications. I was among the first individuals in the country to achieve those certifications that year. I continued my education by participating in environmental testing—air sampling, surface sampling, and bulk sampling, as well as building diagnostics for the facilities mentioned earlier. In 2004, I obtained my Certified Mold Remediator (CMR) certification from the Indoor Air Quality Association (IAQA) and incorporated mold remediation projects following the guidelines set by the American Conference of Governmental Industrial Hygienists (ACGIH), the New York City Department of Health, and the EPA.

I continued improving my ability to understand the entire indoor environment and building envelopes as a multifaceted system while establishing perfect indoor environments for crop production operations. Twenty-four hours a day these environments are monitored to make sure every air quality parameter: temperature, humidity, carbon dioxide levels, particulate control and others, is dialed in to perfection, ensuring the best chance of success. Different rooms throughout these facilities are set up for the different cycles of plant growth. There were rooms set up for propagation, vegetative and flowering, each requiring a different overall environment.

Properly maintaining the HVAC systems and their hygiene required diligent and proactive engagement. It also required properly conducting overall building diagnostics to make sure the entire facility was being maintained and controlled inside and out. This experience not only improved my technical expertise but also deepened my appreciation for the critical role air quality plays in creating healthy environments.

For the last ten years, I have focused on helping individuals and families who are experiencing a negative health reaction when exposed to certain environmental factors within their homes. We've properly diagnosed and resolved many concerning issues: elevated humidity, microbial contamination, negatively pressurized homes, elevated carbon dioxide, extremely high environmental particle count, incorrectly sized HVAC equipment and many others. There's no better feeling than knowing a person's house is no longer an unhealthy environment for them to live in.

Now I'm a licensed HVAC contractor in both California and Florida, with over twenty-five years of hands-on experience addressing indoor air quality concerns. My experience spans the full HVAC system and indoor environment, including temperature and humidity control, particulate control, and a solid understanding of building pressurization and ventilation, each crucial to maintaining clean, comfortable, and safe indoor air. Over the years, I've seen firsthand what solutions work and which ones have fallen short, especially under the relentless Florida heat and humidity, conditions that, when poorly managed, can create dangerously unhealthy indoor environments. My work involves conducting annual inspections to assess how the equipment and indoor environment are handling the challenging, humid climate. This wide-ranging knowledge, combined with decades of practical experience, allows me to provide effective and lasting solutions for homeowners and businesses alike, ensuring healthier indoor spaces and peace of mind.

Chapter 2

What is "Good Indoor Air Quality"?

In recent decades, mold has become a significant concern for homeowners, property managers, and real estate transactions alike. The growing awareness around this issue is due to the potential health and financial impacts that mold contamination can bring. In fact, a 2009 report from the World Health Organization (WHO) estimated that nearly 50% of homes in the United States suffer from excessive dampness and mold growth. Ignoring a mold problem is not just a costly mistake that can result in long-term damage to the property; it can also lead to serious health consequences for the occupants. Mold exposure has been linked to a wide range of allergic reactions and respiratory issues, from mild to severe. Symptoms can include cold and flu-like conditions, chronic fatigue, memory loss, difficulty concentrating, eye irritation, sore or dry throat, skin irritation, sinus infections, and trouble breathing, just to name a few.

Indoor air quality plays a crucial role in the overall health of building occupants, as well as in maintaining building efficiency. Poor indoor air quality can negatively affect human health and productivity, while also contributing to increased energy consumption and operational costs. To mitigate the risk of airborne diseases and contaminants, organizations such as the American Society of Heating, Refrigeration and Air-Conditioning Engineers (ASHRAE) and the Centers for Disease Control (CDC) recommend specific ventilation rates and filtration strategies to maintain healthy indoor air quality. Scientific research underscores the importance of clean air. A noteworthy study conducted by Harvard University's Healthy Buildings Program found that participants performed better on cognitive tests while in an environment with increased ventilation and reduced volatile organic compounds

(VOCs), compared to a standard office setting environment, with some results indicating a boost in cognitive function by up to 100%. This improved air quality could even have an improved impact on significantly reducing the number of sick days taken by individuals suffering from the effects of poor air quality.

Often, poor indoor air quality involves microbial contamination. Mold is a naturally occurring microscopic organism that belongs to the fungi kingdom. Often, the terms "mold" and "fungi" are used interchangeably. In nature, molds play a vital role in breaking down organic material, contributing to the ecosystem's balance. However, when mold takes root in indoor environments, it can pose serious risks. There are numerous types of molds, and people's sensitivity to them varies widely. Some individuals may experience no adverse effects, while others can suffer from significant health problems. Despite widespread concern, there are currently no governmental or industrial regulations that define acceptable levels of mycotoxins or toxigenic mold spores in indoor spaces. This lack of regulatory standards adds another layer of complexity to the challenge of managing indoor air quality effectively.

Molds are challenging. They can infiltrate the body through inhalation, ingestion, and even absorption through the skin, leading to a variety of health issues. For this reason, it is critical to avoid mold exposure whenever possible. Mold growth requires two essential components: a food source and a water source. The food source can be almost anything, including wood, leather, plastic, or cellulose materials, all of which are commonly found in building materials. The water source often occurs from a roof, window, or plumbing leak; however, if the relative humidity (RH) remains at or above 60% for an extended period, the entire environment can become conducive to mold growth.

Under these conditions, mold spores, which are in the air naturally, can extract moisture directly from the air, using condensation nuclei as a source of water. Once the spores land on a surface, whether it's a wall, a piece of furniture, or any other object, they begin to grow, feeding on whatever material is available. During inspections, I have found mold growing in unexpected places, like the paper backing of a picture hanging on a wall. Wood furniture and items like leather belts or shoes become prime buffets for mold in environments with elevated humidity and moisture issues.

Moldy HVAC System Due to Elevated Humidity

One notable case involved a facility that manufactured sonar devices for military submarines. I was there to inspect their HVAC systems and assess the extent of mold contamination, along with providing an estimate for remediation. Mold was clearly visible on the vent covers throughout the building, and the musty smell was overwhelming, reminiscent of a damp gym locker room. My inspection revealed severe microbial contamination not only within the HVAC systems but also throughout the entire facility, all caused by persistent high humidity.

During my inspection, someone in the front office shared their ongoing daily frustration: every morning, they wiped a green, fuzzy growth off their desk, chair, and even wooden pencils, only to find the same growth had returned by the next day. The relative humidity levels throughout the building were consistently between 76% and 82%, creating an ideal environment for mold to flourish.

The root cause of this issue stemmed from an improperly utilized building. The operations of the facility were not aligned with how the HVAC system was intended to function, allowing for continued moisture and enabling mold to spread unchecked. Large bay-style doors that automatically opened and closed to expansive warehouse areas, where there was no air conditioning, further exacerbated the problem. This constant mixing of conditioned and unconditioned, humid air was creating significant challenges for the facility.

I could have cleaned all the HVAC systems, but without addressing the underlying structural issues, it would have been a temporary fix at best. The mold would have quickly returned to the systems. Before any cleaning or remediation could take place, I strongly advised the facility manager to consult with a building engineer to resolve the building's operational design flaws. Only after these systemic problems were corrected would it make sense to clean the HVAC systems. My goal here was to ensure a permanent solution.

Even when humidity levels are controlled, the air handler itself creates an ideal environment for mold growth. Any system designed to provide cool air involves some type of air-handling coil. Inside the air-handling unit, the cooling coil, both while it's cooling and even for some time after it shuts off, operates at 100% relative humidity. This constant moisture allows a biofilm to develop on the aluminum fins of the coil, creating a surface for dirt and mold spores to adhere to, which in turn encourages microbial growth.

A particular concern in these situations is the presence of microbial volatile organic compounds (MVOCs), sometimes referred to as "dirty sock syndrome." This term describes the unpleasant, musty odor that results from the off-gassing of mold as it digests organic materials. The off-gassing of MVOCs includes a wide range of chemical compounds such as alcohols, ketones, aldehydes, esters, carboxylic acids, lactones, terpenes, aromatic hydrocarbons, as well as sulfur and nitrogen compounds. MVOCs are released as byproducts of the metabolic processes of decaying organisms, including fungi, bacteria, and biofilm. The odor can vary depending on concentrations, the type of organic material being consumed, and the presence of other microorganisms. MVOCs are a key indicator of microbial contamination and poor indoor air quality.

Air Handler Contamination

I was hired by a leading eye surgery center to investigate a noxious odor permeating throughout their facility. Upon entering the lobby, I was immediately overwhelmed by the smell of cat urine. Now, just imagine that: patients entering this environment for delicate eye surgery, only to be confronted by an awful and repulsive smell. It was a situation far removed from the standards anyone would expect for a medical procedure, especially one as critical and precise as eye surgery. This odor was a clear sign of a more serious underlying issue that threatened not only the reputation of the facility but also the health and well-being of its patients and staff.

After completing an exhaustive inspection of the HVAC system, it became evident that the source of this offensive odor was microbial contamination that had spread throughout the facility's ductwork and air handling units. Essentially, the HVAC system, particularly the ductwork, had become a delivery system for this foul stench, circulating it from room to room. The extent of the contamination was staggering, with mold colonies flourishing across multiple components of the system. Tackling the root cause of the microbial growth responsible for this persistent odor became my immediate and primary focus.

Discovering and addressing the origin of the mold was the first critical step in resolving the issue. Without identifying the source, any effort to merely eliminate or mask the odor would have been short-lived, and the contamination would quickly return. This understanding of "event occurrence" should always be part of any remediation involving mold issues.

The HVAC system in this facility was large-scale and complex, featuring extensive, internally lined sheet metal ductwork that spanned across multiple levels of the building. These ducts were spacious enough to crawl through, adding another layer of challenges to the remediation process. The air handlers themselves were enormous, comparable in size to a small box truck. Situated behind a large blower wheel and housing was a large flat cooling coil and drain pan. The problems that had led to severe microbial contamination were due to a combination of factors: inadequate equipment maintenance, improper filter replacement schedule, and issues with the condensate drain line.

The system's filters were extremely dirty and clogged, resulting in higher-than-normal static pressure within the HVAC system. This excess pressure prevented the system from functioning optimally. Compounding the issue, the condensate drain line hadn't been properly trapped, which meant that water wasn't draining from the pan as it should have. Instead, it was pooling and stagnating, creating a breeding ground for microbial growth and fostering the development of a nasty muck inside the unit. The large blower wheel, designed to circulate air, was splashing this contaminated water around the unit, sending it straight into the ductwork and throughout the building. It took several months of specialized HVAC remediation to not only deal with the extensive microbial contamination but also to repair the mechanical issues and, ultimately, eliminate the foul odor.

Most air conditioning air handlers are negative pressure cabinets, which means they draw in air from any available opening. Ideally, these cabinets should be tightly sealed to prevent unwanted air infiltration. The condensate drain requires a proper water trap to ensure that humid air isn't being sucked into the system, as that can lead to elevated humidity levels inside the unit, yet another contributor to mold growth. Unfortunately, many systems suffer from mold contamination due to the absence or removal of the water trap, a seemingly small but critical component. When addressing indoor air quality issues related to microbial contamination, controlling humidity and moisture within the HVAC system is essential. Without these controls, mold growth and its associated problems will persist.

According to Bright Hub Engineering, psychrometry is the study of moist air and its various properties, including how to control its temperature, moisture content, or humidity, and how these factors affect both materials and human comfort. This field of study is critical when it comes to understanding thermal comfort, as it provides insight into how air conditions interact with our environment and physical well-being.

To illustrate its importance, consider this example: In Miami, the temperature might be 85 degrees Fahrenheit with a staggering 95% humidity. Under these conditions, the air feels stifling and uncomfortable due to the high moisture content, which hinders the body's ability to cool itself through evaporation. Compare that to San Diego, where the temperature could reach a scorching 115 degrees; but with only 15% humidity. Even though the temperature is significantly higher, the dry air makes it feel far more bearable because the lack of moisture allows sweat to evaporate quickly, cooling the body more efficiently. Here is another example with the same temperature but different humidity levels and what the feel like temperature is.

State	Temperature	Relative Humidity	Feels Like
Tampa	94*	60%	104*
Palm Springs	94*	10%	89*

This contrast highlights how understanding the principles of psychometry can prevent costly mistakes when designing and operating cooling and dehumidification systems for both commercial and residential spaces. Without a solid grasp of how temperature and humidity interact, systems may be improperly calibrated, leading to discomfort for occupants and inefficiency in energy usage. An HVAC system designed with psychrometric principles in mind can ensure that both temperature and humidity are kept at optimal levels, maximizing comfort and minimizing operational costs.

When designing an HVAC system, a properly sized air conditioner is critical in preventing issues such as inadequate cooling, insufficient moisture removal, and unnecessary high electricity costs. When an air conditioning system is too small, it struggles to meet the cooling demands of the indoor space, leaving the environment uncomfortable. On the other hand, an oversized system can cool too quickly without effectively removing humidity, leading to clammy and uncomfortable air. Air conditioning, at its core, involves treating or altering the air by adjusting its temperature or moisture content, depending on the specific requirements of different environments. Today, it's hard to imagine life without this essential piece of equipment, as most people rely on air conditioning daily for their comfort and well-being.

National organizations like ASHRAE (American Society of Heating, Refrigeration, and Air-Conditioning Engineers), NAIMA (North American Insulation Manufacturers Association), NADCA (National Air Duct Cleaners Association), and SMACNA (Sheet Metal and Air Conditioning National Association); provide HVAC codes and standards that establish best practices for the installation and maintenance of air conditioning systems. These standards also address the proper procedures for dealing with microbial contamination within HVAC systems and outline the correct methods for opening, closing, and sealing systems. Ensuring compliance with these codes, standards, and guidelines helps to create efficient, safe, and healthy indoor environments.

Beyond the HVAC industry, agencies such as the Environmental Protection Agency (EPA), the New York City Department of Health, and the American Conference of Governmental Industrial Hygienists (ACGIH) provide additional guidance, particularly when it comes to mold remediation. In 2003, the Institute of Inspection, Cleaning, and Restoration Certification (IICRC) published the ANSI/IICRC S520 Standard for Professional Mold Remediation, which became a critical reference in the industry. This document offers a comprehensive set of guidelines for safely and effectively addressing mold issues in buildings. The IICRC's most recent published Standard, ANSI/IICRC S590 – 2023, Standard for Assessing HVAC Systems Following a

Water, Fire, or Mold Damage Event, contains procedures to perform HVAC assessments and create a written report and Restoration Work Plan (RWP) for residential, commercial, institutional, and healthcare buildings.

Together, these organizations and their standards help professionals navigate a complex industry, one that deals not only with mechanical systems but also with microorganisms that can have a serious negative impact on both human health and the environment. By adhering to these standards, HVAC mold and other remediation professionals can ensure that their work promotes healthier living spaces, greater system efficiency, and reduced environmental risks.

Returning to the original question: What exactly is good indoor air quality? Achieving good indoor air quality involves managing a dynamic and ever-changing environment that requires a delicate balance between the HVAC system, the building envelope, and the human element, which varies widely from person to person. According to the EPA and the National Institute of Occupational Safety and Health (NIOSH) in their "Building Air Quality" guidelines, good indoor air quality is the result of an ongoing interaction among a complex set of factors. Yet, so often, I encounter clients who attempt to improve their air quality by addressing just one factor, inadvertently, in many cases, creating a new problem that worsens their air quality in another way.

To have good indoor air quality, an understanding of what's happening within the indoor environment is critical. This includes knowing how the various components, like the HVAC system, humidity levels, building materials, and even human activity, interact and impact the air being breathed. Monitoring the environment effectively to ensure the cleanest air possible is key. The Occupational Safety and Health Administration

(OSHA) provides a clear framework for what constitutes good indoor air quality: It should include comfortable temperature and humidity levels, an adequate supply of fresh outdoor air, and proper control of pollutants that originate from both inside and outside the building.

However, implementing this ideal balance is not always straightforward, particularly in high-humidity climates. In such environments, even one small misstep, a piece of misguided advice, or the improper installation of equipment, can have a profound and negative impact on the indoor environment, and ultimately, the comfort and health of its occupants. This delicate balance between controlling moisture and particulate, managing airflow, and maintaining system efficiency is what makes the pursuit of good indoor air quality both challenging and critically important.

I attribute our company's success in addressing HVAC mold contamination and indoor air quality challenges to our healthcare-like approach to diagnosing, resolving, verifying, and monitoring both the HVAC system and the indoor environment as a whole, rather than relying on a janitorial or purely surface-level approach. Our objective is not just to remove mold and other contaminants, but to ensure lasting thermal comfort, proper moisture control, and a reduced particle load within the environment. To achieve clean, healthy, and comfortable indoor air quality, the key components to focus on are temperature, moisture, filtration, air purification, and ventilation. Each plays an essential role in maintaining the balance required for optimal air quality.

It's important to understand that there is no one-time quick fix for mold issues and no permanent cure for mold, as it requires ongoing attention through routine inspections and proper maintenance. The key to success in this field is not just immediate remediation but the development of comprehensive, ongoing plans to ensure that mold and poor indoor air quality issues do not return.

Any remediation attempt that doesn't include long-term plans

to maintain systems and prevent recurrence

is short-sighted and destined to fail.

– American Conference of Governmental Industrial Hygienists

Chapter 3

Molds Commonly Found in HVAC Systems

There are several types of molds commonly found, and a few that are not so common within HVAC systems. After reviewing thousands of environmental assessment reports, I've identified some frequent and unwelcome visitors that seem to show up repeatedly. While the following are just a few of the most common, many other molds can and do make their presence known. When mold is suspected in an HVAC system, a surface sample can determine species. Air sampling is also valuable for assessing the broader environmental impact, but it has limitations when it comes to pinpointing molds, specifically within HVAC systems.

Here are several molds that are frequently found in HVAC systems:

Cladosporium – One of the most commonly encountered molds, Cladosporium has approximately 500 species, though only about 20 are regularly found in indoor environments. This fungus can lead to skin lesions, nail fungus, sinusitis, asthma, and pulmonary infections. Its spores are light and easily aerosolized, making them quick to spread through the air. Often found in dirty air conditioning systems, especially in condensation reservoirs, Cladosporium can sporulate heavily, making it one of the most significant fungal allergens affecting airways. Its colonies typically appear as powdery or velvety patches, ranging from olive-green to olive-brown in color.

Aspergillus – With over 182 species, sixteen of which are known to cause human diseases, Aspergillus is another frequently encountered mold. Aspergillosis, an infection caused by this mold, is the second most common fungal infection requiring hospitalization in the U.S. Many Aspergillus species are allergenic and produce mycotoxins that may be harmful to humans.

Penicillium – Easily aerosolized, Penicillium is often found in materials like cellulose, carpet, wallpaper, and fiberglass duct insulation. Of the 225 species of Penicillium, around 70 are frequently encountered in indoor environments. This mold is known to cause allergic reactions and can lead to conditions such as hypersensitivity pneumonitis. Some species of Penicillium are also capable of producing mycotoxins. It has been found growing on surfaces like painted walls, wooden boards, and wallpaper.

Hyphal Fragments – These fragments are present wherever fungal spores exist. Falling under the bioaerosols category, hyphal fragments are tiny airborne particles derived from living organisms like mold. These particles can contribute to allergies and other health issues.

Rust – Microbial corrosion, or biocorrosion, is a type of corrosion influenced by the presence and activity of microorganisms in biofilms that form on corroding materials. Microbiologically induced corrosion (MIC) can significantly damage metal surfaces, causing them to deteriorate. In HVAC systems, rust can lead to equipment malfunction and failure, as pitted surfaces impair functionality.

Bacteria – Among the earliest life forms on Earth, bacteria are single-cell organisms that are omnipresent in various environments. While they lack a specific transport mechanism, bacteria can attach themselves to tiny airborne particles, allowing them to be distributed throughout an indoor environment.

Mycotoxins – These naturally occurring toxic compounds are produced by certain types of molds. Mycotoxins can cause a variety of health problems, with some individuals being more affected than others. Their impact depends on the specific type of mold, the dose of exposure, and the route of exposure, whether through inhalation, skin contact, or ingestion. Hundreds of mycotoxins have been identified, but the most concerning for human health are aflatoxins and Ochratoxin A. According to WHO, these are among the most poisonous and are produced by certain molds like Aspergillus flavus, Aspergillus parasiticus, and Penicillium. Air sampling has many limitations in detecting mycotoxins so detection should be done through bulk, surface, or dust sampling like an Environmental Relative Moldiness Index (ERMI).

In addition to the commonly found molds, there are a few that are less frequently encountered in HVAC systems, but they do appear from time to time during swab tests of the system's internal components. These molds include:

Stachybotrys – Often dubbed "black mold" or "toxic mold" by the media, Stachybotrys Chartarum thrives in water-damaged, cellulose-rich materials such as sheetrock, paper, ceiling tiles, and wallpaper. This mold is particularly hazardous due to its ability to produce potent mycotoxins. Exposure to Stachybotrys can occur through inhalation, ingestion, or skin contact, leading to symptoms like burning sensations in the mouth and nasal passages, cold and flu-like symptoms, headaches, and fever.

Chaetomium – Growing in similar conditions to Stachybotrys, Chaetomium is sometimes referred to as the "other black mold." It is also highly toxic, producing large quantities of mycotoxins. This mold can cause skin and nail infections, cerebral infections, allergic reactions, and asthma. Other symptoms of exposure may include coughing, memory loss, nosebleeds, seizures, dermatitis, fever, and internal lesions.

Fusarium – Requiring extremely wet conditions, Fusarium is often found in walls with prolonged water intrusion. It can lead to hay fever or asthma-like symptoms.

Memnoniella – A close relative of Stachybotrys, Memnoniella is a mycotoxin-producing mold that typically grows on water-damaged construction materials like wet gypsum board, particularly in warm, humid climates. It can also be found on composite wood and ceiling tiles.

No matter the species of mold, it's crucial to identify and address the underlying cause of microbial growth before proceeding with remediation. Proper mold remediation must follow stringent protocols to ensure the safety of the environment and its occupants. While it may be tempting to rely on DIY methods or YouTube tutorials, this can be extremely dangerous. Seeking assistance from licensed and certified professionals is always the safest and most effective route when dealing with mold contamination in HVAC systems or the overall environment.

Chapter 4

Types of Heating and Cooling Systems

There are many different types of HVAC systems, each suited to specific environments based on factors such as climate, geography, and the particular heating and cooling needs of the area, whether it be humid, dry, or somewhere in between. In this chapter, I'll focus on a few common systems designed for residential and light commercial applications, which most people are likely familiar with. Large-scale commercial and industrial systems, however, are complex enough to warrant their own dedication, perhaps in another book.

Central Air Conditioning Systems

Often referred to as a split system, this is one of the most popular choices for homes and businesses due to its flexibility and adaptability. It can be configured to meet the specific cooling and heating demands of an entire building. A central air conditioning system is a forced-air setup where the condenser is located outside, while the air handler can be situated inside the home, under the house, in the attic, or in the garage. Ductwork is attached to both the intake and exhaust sides of the air handler. The intake ducts bring air to the unit for conditioning (filtering, heating, and/or cooling), while the exhaust ducts return the conditioned air to the living space.

Central air systems cool all rooms at once, using the ductwork to distribute air throughout the building. Three simple and common types of split systems are straight cool systems, heat pump systems, and furnace systems. All three systems share the cooling function via a cooling coil, but they differ in their heating methods. The straight cool system relies on an electric heat strip for warmth. Heat pump systems reverse the refrigerant flow in the outdoor unit to generate heat and often have an electric heat strip for backup. Furnace systems use natural gas burners for heating and a cooling coil for air conditioning.

One of the key advantages of central air conditioning is that these systems can be disassembled, allowing for proper cleaning and maintenance. Additionally, various air quality improvement technologies can be integrated into these systems, such as UV light assemblies, induct air purifiers, advanced filtration systems, as well as ventilation and dehumidification equipment.

Package Units

Similar to split systems in functionality, package units contain all the components: condenser, air handler, and more, inside a single cabinet. These units are installed outside the building, and ductwork usually runs under the house or through the wall to distribute conditioned air. Package units are common in both residential and commercial settings. In commercial applications, these are often called rooftop units (RTUs) as they sit on the roof, with ductwork running down into the building. While package units can be taken apart for cleaning, extra care must be taken to ensure that the air handling cabinet is properly sealed, especially since the entire unit is exposed to the elements.

Ductless Mini-Splits

According to the Air-Conditioning, Heating, and Refrigeration Institute (AHRI), ductless mini-split systems consist of an outdoor unit and an indoor air handler mounted in the room, which directly blows cooled air into that space. These systems are ideal for small areas such as workshops or room additions where installing ductwork may not be practical. Recent advancements have enabled mini-spits systems to provide cooling to multiple rooms without the need for ductwork, making them increasingly popular. While not as robust as central air systems, they excel in their intended applications and provide a convenient solution for certain situations.

Evaporative Coolers

Also known as swamp coolers, evaporative coolers are an energy-efficient and natural method for cooling indoor air. These systems are particularly effective in hot, dry climates where humidity levels are low. They work by passing air through a moist pad, which cools the air before circulating it through the home using a fan. However, these systems are unsuitable for humid climates, as they introduce additional moisture into the air, which can exacerbate humidity problems.

Window Air Conditioners

One of the most common types of air conditioners, window units are a popular choice for cooling single rooms or small areas. These units operate similarly to package systems, with all components, condenser, evaporator, and fan, housed within a single enclosure. Most window air conditioners come equipped with a washable filter, although these filters tend to be less efficient than those found in larger systems. If microbial contamination is a concern, it is generally recommended to replace the entire unit rather than attempt remediation of the equipment due to the cost.

Portable Air Conditioners

Like window units, portable air conditioners contain all their components within a single enclosure. Their key advantage is mobility, allowing users to move the unit from room to room as needed. These systems also typically have washable filters, but if there is concern about microbial contamination, replacement of the unit is advised.

Cooling Tower Systems

While primarily reserved for large commercial and industrial applications, it's worth mentioning that cooling towers are part of more complex HVAC systems. These systems often utilize variable air volume (VAV), constant air volume (CAV), and fan coil units (FCUs), which act as small air handlers to serve different zones within a building.

In conclusion, the diversity of HVAC systems reflects the varying needs of different environments and building types. Each system has its strengths and ideal applications, whether it's for a small residential space, a commercial office, or an industrial plant. Understanding these systems and their proper maintenance is essential to ensuring that the indoor environment remains comfortable, efficient, and healthy.

Chapter 5

Parts of the Residential HVAC System Explained

To simplify things, the typical residential HVAC system can be broken down into three primary areas for hygiene and maintenance: the return side, the air handling unit, and the supply side. The air is returned to the air handler to be conditioned and then supplied to the indoor space. Returned, conditioned, supplied. Here's a quick guide to understanding these key components:

Return Ductwork – The return ductwork pulls air from the indoor environment and brings it back to the air handler, where it is filtered, heated, or cooled. Return ductwork usually has a return plenum connected to the air handler, a trunkline, and maybe branch runs that connect the return plenum to the ceiling, wall, and/or floor grill. In some cases, the filter is placed at these openings using what is known as a filter-backed grill, and in other cases, the filter is placed prior to the air handler in the filter rack.

Not all systems use conventional materials for dedicated return ductwork. Some systems use the open space above drop ceilings or concrete walls under buildings for air returns, and high-rise buildings often use wall cavities to return air to the HVAC system. In some configurations, such as an air handler sitting on a stand in a closet, the air is drawn into the system from the open room, known as an open-air return system. Closing doors can change the pressurization within the space unless jumpers allow air to move from one space to another. Even without ductwork, air is still returned to the system to be conditioned. In this case, the filter is usually installed in the filter rack prior to the air entering the air handler coil.

Air Handler – The air handler is responsible for conditioning the air. It filters, heats, or cools the air depending on the system's settings. In cooling mode, the refrigeration process also dehumidifies the air to some extent as moisture is removed from the air. This moisture condenses on the coil fins and runs down into the drain pan, eventually making its way outside via the drain line. The filter, usually located at the leading edge of the air handler cabinet, cleans the air before it enters the air handling unit. The filter can be installed in a rack at the air handler or in the return grill located in the ceiling, wall, or sometimes the floor.

Supply Ductwork – The supply ductwork delivers the conditioned air from the air handler back into the living space. This air is filtered, cooled, and/or heated, and then circulated back into the environment. This cycle repeats until the system turns off. Like the return ductwork, supply ductwork usually includes a supply plenum, which is connected to the air handler cabinet, a main trunkline, junction boxes, branch runs, boot boxes, and vent covers. The ductwork can be made of various materials, including flexible duct (flex duct), fiberboard (also called duct board), externally wrapped sheet metal, or internally lined sheet metal.

Like any HVAC component, the correct installation and regular maintenance of ductwork are essential for maintaining indoor air quality and ensuring the system functions efficiently. NADCA recommends inspecting HVAC systems once a year, and in some cases, every six months, depending on the building's classification and needs. An inspection schedule should be tailored to each environmental and individual situation.

Ductwork Types:

Flex Ductwork – Introduced in the early 1970s, flex duct is a versatile option resembling a slinky, typically sold in 25-foot sections. It consists of a polymeric inner film (the air barrier), insulation wrapped around it (the thermal barrier), and a silver mylar jacket to hold everything together. In crawl spaces, flex ducts often have a thicker black cover for extra protection. Flex ductwork is ideal for navigating awkward spaces, corners, and tight spots where rigid ductwork wouldn't fit. Energy codes usually require an R6 insulating value for flex ducts, but in some cases, R8 could be required or necessary.

There are many reasons to clean flexible ductwork, and when done correctly can be very beneficial. However, in the case of microbial contamination, this type of duct surface cannot be effectively cleaned and should be replaced. Proper engineering controls should be implemented during the removal of contaminated ductwork.

Fiberboard (Duct Board) – Fiberboard, or duct board, is semi-rigid compressed fiberglass insulation used in residential and light commercial systems. It's commonly used to create plenums and junction boxes where a flex duct is attached using connecting collars. Its porous surface means cleaning may be limited depending on the type and level of contamination.

Client's Comment: "I was told this type of ductwork can't be cleaned."

My Response: "Wow, I wonder where they got that information?" I then show the client NAIMA's publication on Cleaning Fibrous Glass Insulated Air Duct Systems, which outlines recommended practices for cleaning duct board, even with rotating brushes, when done properly. Most of the time, this duct surface is cleaned using a method known as contact vacuuming.

A round nylon brush and HEPA vacuum are used to remove non-adhered substances from the duct surface. However, if microbial contamination or odors are present, cleaning alone may not be enough to pass a clearance test. After cleaning the duct surface, an HVAC resurfacing coating product can be applied, albeit cautiously. The main purpose of coating a porous duct surface is to lock down loose or fraying materials, and in some cases, to reduce fiber erosion. Regardless of the type of ductwork, if there is microbial contamination, replacement should be the first consideration and recommendation.

Internally Lined Sheet Metal – This type of ductwork has an exterior made of sheet metal and an interior lined with insulation, making it a porous surface like duct board. Sometimes, only the first few feet of ductwork are internally lined for sound absorption, while the rest is externally wrapped. This type of ductwork is common in large commercial buildings and can be cleaned. In cases of odors or microbial staining, an HVAC coating product may be necessary, or relining the damaged duct may also be an option, though it can be challenging in difficult-to-reach areas. In many large commercial applications, the ductwork has been installed in such a manner that replacing it isn't an option. This is when repair, remediation, and restoration will have to be considered and performed.

Externally Wrapped Sheet Metal – In this system, the interior surface is metal, while insulation is wrapped around the outside. This non-porous surface can be cleaned and disinfected, though accessing all surface areas for cleaning may be challenging due to limited space and the presence of turning vanes. Closing and sealing the ductwork to prevent air leakage and ensure proper system operation also requires specialized training.

Air Handler

The air conditioning system is often one of the most expensive pieces of equipment a homeowner has. Adding the duct system significantly increases that investment. Routine maintenance helps extend the life of the equipment and ensures clean air delivery to the home. Air handlers vary widely, from window units and mini splits to package units and central air systems. Large commercial systems often use cooling towers and distribute conditioned air through variable air volume (VAV), constant air volume (CAV), or fan coil units (FCUs).

For now, we'll focus on central air conditioning systems, which are versatile and customizable. These systems are ideal for integrating emerging air quality technologies. When a central air conditioning system isn't being used, there are other alternatives, like stand-alone dehumidifiers and air purifiers, to achieve improved indoor air quality.

Inside the air handler cabinet, you'll find the evaporator coil (cooling coil), drain pan, and blower assembly (which includes the blower housing, wheel, and motor). The cabinet typically includes a 1" filter rack, an electric heating strip, and insulation lining. The cabinet also contains wiring, transformers, fan relays, capacitors, and maybe a

43

control board. To properly clean the unit, the blower assembly and the cooling coil/drain pan will need to be removed.

The refrigerant is pumped into the compressor and stored, allowing the cooling coil to be removed for cleaning. Specialized cleaning products designed for HVAC systems must be used. Consideration of the client's sensitivity to certain solutions and products, whether natural or not, must be understood. The blower assembly is also removed, disassembled, and cleaned, ensuring the motor stays dry. With all the components removed, there is full access to the inside of the cabinet so that the surface of the liner can be addressed.

The cabinet's insulation acts as a thermal barrier. Depending on its condition, the insulation can be cleaned or replaced. In cases with mold contamination or a damaged or deteriorated liner, the insulation can be removed, the surface cleaned, and then it can be relined with a closed cell liner. This type of insulation is a polymer foam insulation that is waterproof and cleanable.

Air Handler Location

The air handler can be installed in various locations, such as horizontally in the attic, garage or under the house, or vertically in a closet or garage. Package units are typically located outside the house. The location usually depends on the house's framing and the layout needed for efficient ductwork distribution. If you want some additional square footage or that extra-large walk-in closet, for example, having the air handler somewhere other than in the house is usually the option.

Client's Question: "Where's the best place for the air handler to be installed to prevent mold?"

The answer is: No location can completely prevent mold. In my experience, I've found mold contamination in air handlers installed in every conceivable location. The key problem is often not the location itself but rather results from other factors like poor sealing around access panels, refrigerant lines, and filter racks, as well as un-trapped drain lines, all allowing humid, unconditioned air to enter the system. Improperly installed or sealed ductwork can also lead to pressurization problems, contributing to elevated humidity and mold growth.

Other issues include improperly sized units or restrictive filters that cause air to bypass the filter and allow unfiltered air to enter the system. This added restriction can increase static pressure and lead to moisture buildup in the unit. Outdoor air intake ducts can introduce humidity, increasing the risk of microbial growth if the air isn't properly dehumidified before entering the system.

Water issues are also a major concern. Air handlers are prone to leaking water from clogged condensate lines or frozen coils that can form blocks of ice and later melt, causing water damage. Water, condensation, and moisture must be controlled. If the air conditioner setpoint is so low that the unit never shuts off, this can cause the air handler cabinet to become so cold it reaches the dew point. At dew point, condensation will form on the cabinet and can run down onto the wood platform causing staining and possibly other water event issues.

Regardless of the location, proper installation, sealing, operation, and maintenance are crucial to preventing issues with water, humidity, and air quality. When air handlers are installed inside the house, additional measures like safety drain pans, water alarms, and emergency shut-off switches can help prevent water from damaging the home. Even if everything is correctly installed and operating, air handlers have water issues. In the summertime, the evaporator coil can produce about one gallon of water an hour, which is sent out of the drain line. If the air handler is located inside the house and the drain line clogs, this water can quickly damage interior walls and ceilings.

When considering trying to move an air handler from its original location, the framing of the house can sometimes present challenges. There must be enough room, not only for the air handler; but also for the ductwork (supply and return) that will run to and from the cabinet. Additional space is also required to perform the work. This relocation of the equipment requires the installation of new refrigerant lines, thermostat wires, and a drain line. Finally, an electrician may be necessary to move the main power line to the equipment.

In summary, regardless of the air handler's location, proper installation and upkeep of it and associated ductwork are essential in maintaining a healthy, efficient system. Proper building pressurization, humidity control, filter selection, and maintenance are critical to preventing mold growth and ensuring the system operates smoothly. Always seek out a licensed and qualified company that understands all these different parameters and how they need to function cohesively for the best results.

Chapter 6

Diagnosing the HVAC System for Mold

In 2020, the global pandemic spurred a surge in companies claiming to be indoor air quality "experts", but far from professionals, most lacking the proper qualifications and knowledge to do the right job. Unfortunately, most of these opportunistic companies fail to achieve the results expected by clients suffering from microbial contamination in their HVAC systems. They often believe that simply cleaning and sanitizing mold out of duct systems is sufficient, which couldn't be further from the truth. Too often, homeowners find themselves at their wit's end due to ineffective work from previous AC and cleaning companies who are offering band-aide solutions and aren't addressing the broader environmental factors.

Here is an analogy: Fast Food vs. Nutritionist — The traditional HVAC service companies are like fast food chains, quick to provide what's convenient and readily available for the immediate need. In contrast, we are like a nutritionist who tailors plans based on the specific health needs of clients, focusing on wellness and long-term benefits. We aren't just "serving up" air conditioning; we are carefully crafting environments where people can breathe cleaner, healthier air.

The typical AC or cleaning company isn't an inspection service company. Over the years I have come to realize that this is who most people call to help fix serious indoor air quality issues that are negatively affecting one's health. Without any types of medical certifications or licenses, companies are offering services that make claims of environmental improvements that will allow someone to feel healthier. A quick free estimate will not include the time it takes to accurately diagnose and resolve problems that could be causing serious health issues, and I certainly don't know anyone who is investigating, diagnosing, and resolving indoor air quality problems for free. Remember:

Free advice is worth every penny you are paying for it.

-Matthew Etzler

Having a qualified and experienced professional to inspect and assess the HVAC system and its impact on the indoor environment is essential. According to NADCA, at a minimum, this individual should have a verifiable working knowledge of basic HVAC system design, fundamental engineering practices, current HVAC cleaning and restoration techniques, and applicable industry standards. Many states require companies to hold a state air conditioning contractor's license to perform any HVAC-related assessment and/or work, whether mechanical or hygienic (cleaning). Ask for the contractor's license number and verify it through the state licensing portal. A referred or recommended company is always a good place to start.

When recommendations are made to clean, remediate, or replace ductwork and AC equipment without addressing possible underlying issues such as poor installation, ventilation, insulation, or pressurization problems, the system and the indoor environment will continue to struggle. A thorough inspection must evaluate not only the mechanical and hygiene aspects of the HVAC system but also the surrounding environment to determine if it is negatively affecting the HVAC system's ability to function as intended.

The first and most critical step is to identify the air quality issues the HVAC system may be causing, as well as any other areas of concern within the overall environment. For example, one common environmental factor that can cause issues to a properly installed HVAC system is the use of spray foam insulation, which, while effective in sealing and insulating, can trap moisture in humid climates. This insulation is acceptable to use; however, it does require proper humidity control to avoid moisture and mold problems not only in the attic space but within the home as well.

We have completed many projects where spray foam insulation was installed. One recent project with this type of insulation was causing the humidity in the attic to soar close to 90% while the indoor humidity was in the mid-seventies, even with standalone dehumidifiers running. The air handler and ductwork were contaminated with microbial growth, and a musty odor permeated the attic. The rafters were damp to the touch, and water dripped from the spray foam insulation onto the ceiling. Water stains on the ceiling were visible throughout the building, and the drywall was so soft that our wall saw couldn't cut through it properly.

Sometimes moisture problems in the attic are caused by insufficient ventilation. This can happen when a new roof is installed, but the ridge vent isn't reopened, or ventilation holes are blocked. Sometimes, additional insulation added to the attic for energy efficiency ends up blocking soffits, further restricting airflow. Increasing the R-value of the insulation in the attic can change the heat load within the house. This could cause the air conditioner to operate less during cooling cycles, and elevated humidity is usually the result.

Issues stemming from improperly installed or incorrectly sized HVAC systems can lead to mold growth not only within the system but also throughout the entire indoor environment. That's why it's crucial to have the AC system, ductwork and its surroundings properly inspected and investigated. Merely cleaning or replacing equipment and ductwork won't resolve the overall indoor air quality problem if the root cause, or in most cases, causes are not identified.

Client's Question: "We paid for a home inspection. Why didn't the home inspector's report indicate that there was a severe problem with the air conditioning system being contaminated with mold? We probably wouldn't have bought the house if we knew how bad it was."

This is a common misconception. Home inspections performed as part of most real estate transactions only assess the basic mechanical functions of the HVAC system, whether it heats or cools, and provides minor visual remarks on its exterior condition. Home inspectors are not qualified to assess the overall mechanical or hygiene conditions of the system. The detailed inspection of the air conditioner homeowners think they are getting can only be conducted by a licensed air conditioning contractor, ideally one with experience in dealing with microbial contamination.

Client: "I had a mold assessment done for my house and the assessors report has protocols for addressing the environment which includes cleaning and sanitizing the ductwork. How much do you charge to do this?"

Most mold assessment companies will mention the HVAC system in their reports, directing their clients to consult with a licensed AC contractor and NADCA certified company to completely inspect the HVAC system. Even if the mold remediation company is really trying to help someone, recommendations made regarding the cleaning, remediation or replacement of the HVAC system should be received cautiously. The inspection of the HVAC system should include the hygiene of the system, proper installation of the AC equipment and ductwork, and the mechanical functioning's of the equipment. Determining if a whole home dehumidifier or filtration system can be installed takes careful consideration. Getting this part right is very important to achieve an overall cleaner environment. There are many times that the system can be cleaned and remediated, but ensuring the current situation doesn't quickly return requires a much more detailed inspection.

Proper inspection involves opening and accessing various areas of the ductwork, which must then be resealed with appropriate materials. The mechanical functioning's of the system should be evaluated to ensure the equipment is operating properly and isn't causing any problems. In some cases, this inspection may recommend environmental testing to determine what type of mold, if any, is present. Other times, areas outside of the HVAC system may require additional investigation to check for plumbing or roof leaks, improperly installed windows and other structural defects that can cause water damage. Understanding the pressurization dynamics of the home or business is also crucial in controlling humidity and preventing other airborne contaminants from entering the indoor space. Diagnosing what could cause someone to feel ill in their home or workplace is a serious matter that requires careful consideration of all factors.

During the inspection, a licensed AC contractor and Certified Ventilation Inspector (CVI) will inspect the HVAC system, using tools such as service gauges, moisture meters, thermal imaging cameras, camera scopes, anemometers for airflow measurements, manometers for static pressure checks, and temperature and humidity meters. Depending on the individual's health concerns and the environment, additional building investigation, testing and/or sampling may be required.

Within the HVAC system, surface sampling may be needed to determine the species of mold that is present. Outside the system, surface and air sampling can be conducted, along with the Environmental Relative Moldiness Index (ERMI) test, which was released by the EPA in 2006. This test uses PCR analysis to detect fungal DNA in surface dust, providing a record of what has been circulating in the air. A normal ERMI score is below 2. According to Dr.

Ritchie Shoemaker, a medical doctor and world authority on mold assessment and treatment, individuals experiencing adverse health effects from microbial exposure, particularly those with Chronic Inflammatory Response Syndrome (CIRS), should avoid further exposure as the first step in their treatment.

Identifying the conditions that contribute to microbial growth is one of the most critical first steps in the remediation process. Without this clear understanding of the events or building dynamics responsible for microbial growth, no effective control strategy can be implemented (ACGIH). This requires intricate investigation and testing by qualified individuals. In most cases, all the issues within the environment will need to be addressed to attain improved or optimal indoor air quality. When more than just the HVAC system needs to be assessed, it is important to find a knowledgeable, Certified Mold Assessment company to provide inspection and testing of the environment. When you combine the environmental assessment report, provided by the mold assessment company, with the HVAC inspection and environmental impact assessment report, you have an all-inclusive understanding of what is occurring within the environment, why it's occurring, and procedures on properly addressing any deficiencies.

I know I keep repeating myself, but I can't stress enough the importance of finding a qualified professional who truly understands the HVAC system, its impact on the entire environment and the diagnostic process. Once the HVAC system and its surrounding areas have been properly evaluated, this person should be able to clearly explain the deficiencies, their underlying causes, and what the corrective measures are. When necessary, they should be able to collaborate with the environmental mold assessment and testing company to make sure the entire environment is properly addressed. The next critical step is to develop a scope of work and safety protocols for resolving these issues, followed by verification measures to ensure the corrections are successful and sustainable.

To conclude, properly diagnosing an HVAC system and indoor environment for mold shouldn't be a one-size-fits-all approach. It requires a combination of expertise, specialized tools, and a deep understanding of both the mechanical and environmental factors involved. With a comprehensive evaluation and a well-thought-out remediation plan, significant improvements in indoor air quality can be achieved, leading to a healthier living and working environment.

Chapter 7

Cleaning and Sanitizing Moldy Ductwork

I'll say it again, air duct cleaning is a great service when it's done properly, but let's be clear about air duct cleaning and moldy ductwork, especially flex duct:

Moldy flex ductwork cannot be successfully cleaned and should be replaced.

You also can't simply fog mold out of the ductwork. There are acceptable restoration options for other duct types, but the limitations should be disclosed and completely understood. When companies claim they can clean and sanitize moldy ductwork, they often endanger the occupants by doing the wrong thing. What may seem like a quick fix doesn't eliminate the mold or solve the problem.

Is there a standard explaining how to properly apply sanitizers or fogging agents to ductwork with claims of killing and eliminating mold? The short answer is no. There is no industry standard or protocol that outlines the proper method for sanitizing ductwork, particularly in the context of eliminating mold. Be wary of companies claiming their products are "EPA-approved" for this purpose. The product must be registered and not just approved for the intended purpose. The truth is that while a product may be EPA registered, this registration only means that the product has been tested for specific uses, which must be clearly stated. Don't be fooled by the "EPA-approved" tactic. Always ask for documentation showing the specific intended use of any product, especially for mold remediation claims in air ducts.

Sanitizers, as defined by the EPA, are classified as pesticides, and their registered use is to reduce, but not necessarily eliminate, bacteria on inanimate surfaces to levels deemed acceptable by public health standards. In general, sanitizers are effective only against bacteria.

Some sanitizers may also be registered for use in treating mold, but the label must clearly indicate that they are safe and effective for use in air ducts specifically. If you're concerned about sanitizers or other cleaning products, the EPA and Antimicrobial Division websites are good resources to learn more about sanitizers, deodorizers, disinfectants, and HVAC resurfacing or coating products.

The EPA has made it clear that the application of chemical biocides to kill bacteria and fungi in HVAC systems can be appropriate under certain conditions, but research has not demonstrated their effectiveness in duct cleaning. Moreover, the EPA warns that biocides have not been proven to be safe for use in ductwork, and none have been approved for the purpose of eliminating mold from air ducts.

Client's Question: "What about companies offering a 'green technology fog' that promises to eliminate all the mold from the ductwork and air handling unit? One company even claimed it would 'explode the mold away.'"

The truth is, there is no standard for fogging ventilation ductwork to eliminate mold. Any company making such claims is simply fabricating the effectiveness of their method. Offering a service to address mold problems without adhering to any kind of industry standards, especially in a health-related context, is negligent and potentially dangerous. If they were in the health care industry, it would be considered malpractice. Companies offering these "green fogging" solutions often can't explain key details, such as the method of application, the dosage rate, the target organism, how frequently the application should be made, or the timing necessary for achieving effective results. While these companies promise a fast and inexpensive fix, the reality is that fogging ductwork won't resolve the problem. Never allow anyone to fog the HVAC system with claims that the product will magically eliminate mold.

This approach has been proven ineffective through post-testing. After these companies fog the ductwork, the mold is still there; it doesn't just disappear. Moreover, they often fail to address the underlying cause of the mold growth, leaving the door open for a repeat problem. In my opinion, these companies are the modern-day snake oil salesmen. Heed caution. If there is microbial growth present, it usually indicates a deeper problem within the air conditioning system or overall environment, and that problem must be addressed to prevent future issues.

Client's Question: "If you can't replace the ductwork because of mold contamination, isn't it better to try cleaning and fogging it rather than doing nothing?"

Mold can't be fogged out of ductwork. There are duct types that can be restored, but flex isn't one of them. When visible mold (Condition 3) is found on flex ductwork, it's not cleanable. Attempting to clean it can stir up the mold, making the air quality far worse. Disturbing mold on flex ductwork, such as running a rotating brush over it, can cause the mold to release spores into the air as a defense mechanism. Some mold may be vacuumed up, but most will remain adhered to the duct surface. Worse, if the environmental conditions that caused the mold aren't addressed, the mold will continue to grow unabated.

There is an acceptable remediation process for several other duct types if it's thoroughly explained and the limitations understood. If the ductwork is duct board or fiberboard, this porous type of ductwork can be HEPA vacuumed. The surface is cleaned, known as contact vacuuming, using a round nylon brush. The surface will be cleaned of any chunky, non-adhered substances, but the surface will still be contaminated. Cleaning mold from ductwork is comparable to HVAC fire restoration. We can vacuum the soot out of the ductwork, but we can't suck the smoke odor out. Restoration occurs when the application of an HVAC approved coating/resurfacing product is applied. The duct surface is no longer exposed to any air passing through the duct. In other words, it has been restored. There are many occasions when this really is the only option. In some cases, the ductwork isn't accessible for replacement, and in others, it's just budgetary.

Internally lined sheet metal ductwork is like duct board in that the insulation inside the ductwork exposed to the air is porous. This type of ductwork is more challenging to access, but once inside, it's treated the same as duct board. The other type of ductwork is externally wrapped sheet metal, where the inside of the ductwork exposed to the air is non-porous metal. Many access openings are required to clean and properly decontaminate sheet metal ductwork. When cleaning large commercial systems, often, the technician will crawl through the ductwork to prevent timely opening, closing, and sealing of the duct access holes.

Most sheet metal ductwork uses turning vanes where the duct makes ninety-degree turns. Access into the duct is necessary on both sides of the turning vane. Opening and closing sheet metal ductwork is time-consuming, and the cost for this type of work is more expensive. It gets tricky when the sheet metal ductwork is in a house attic space, and most of it isn't accessible. If you can't properly open and close the ductwork, the entire system probably isn't being cleaned. Vent covers need to be removed, air handlers need to be opened, and access into the supply plenum, main trunkline, and junction boxes is necessary to clean the entire system. We wouldn't brush only half our teeth. Why would attempting to clean only half of the HVAC system be acceptable?

To sum it up, moldy ductwork, especially flex ductwork, should be replaced, not cleaned. Efforts to fog or sanitize mold out of ductwork are not effective, and they won't solve the underlying problem that caused mold to grow in the first place. The best solution is always to identify and correct the underlying causes of mold growth; and then replace any affected ductwork to ensure a healthy indoor environment. Any part of the HVAC system that is cleaned or remediated should have a verification process in place as part of the overall corrective action plan.

Chapter 8

The Scope of Work

Once the HVAC inspection and environmental impact assessment are completed, the next step is to create a Scope of Work (SOW). This document is critical for outlining the specific expectations, tasks, and objectives of the project. It serves as a roadmap for transforming the HVAC system and environment from its current state to a healthy, clean, and functional system. The SOW is a formal guide that provides structure and clarity for the entire project.

The SOW should include not only the tasks to be performed but also the objectives that will resolve the issues identified during the inspection. It must clearly detail how the project will progress, addressing safety protocols, containment strategies, and any other relevant information specific to the project. Safety protocols are especially important in projects involving mold remediation or hazardous environmental factors. This ensures that both the workers and the occupants are protected throughout the process.

A strong communication plan is essential and should be outlined in the SOW. This plan specifies who will be responsible for communicating during the project, how often updates will be provided, and which methods of communication are acceptable, whether that's through phone calls, text messages, or emails. It's crucial that everyone involved knows who to contact and how to stay informed about the project's progress. Any additional details pertinent to the project should also be included to avoid misunderstanding or delays.

In the HVAC industry, when ductwork is replaced, it is generally replaced size for size, with the configuration remaining largely the same. The only time the size or configuration changes is when a heat load calculation reveals the need for something different or when specific modifications like replacing square sheet metal ductwork with round flex ductwork are required. Proper sizing and configuration are crucial to ensure the HVAC system operates efficiently, maintaining comfort in the indoor space.

The SOW should be explicit about which components of the air duct system will be replaced and which will remain. For instance, the supply duct system consists of various parts such as the plenum, trunkline, junction boxes, branch runs, boot boxes, and vent covers. Not every part always requires replacement. Sometimes, only the flex ductwork needs to be replaced, in which case the job is listed on the permit as a partial air duct replacement. Any components that are not replaced must be cleaned, remediated, and/or restored to Condition 1 (normal fungal ecology). All limitations and decisions should be well-documented and agreed upon, particularly when anything less than a full system replacement is considered in the presence of mold contamination.

As you can see, the SOW can be quite detailed, but more importantly, it must be informative. According to NADCA, the scope of work should include, but is not limited to, the following:

1. Clearly identify which HVAC components will be cleaned, restored, or replaced.

2. Detailing the environmental engineering controls required for the specific project.

3. Outlining the cleaning, restoration, or replacement protocols to be used, tailored to the specific needs of the project.

4. Identifying any additional trades involved and their respective tasks.

5. A project schedule, including start dates, estimated completion times, and any important milestones.

6. A communication plan that lists company names, contact details, and the responsibilities of everyone involved.

7. Submittals such as Safety Data Sheets (SDS) for any products being used, along with photo documentation when required.

8. Engineering controls to protect both workers and occupants from chemical vapors and odors.

Depending on the building classification or specific conditions, the SOW can also include the following additional items:

1. Outline of the client's responsibilities during the project.

2. Information on necessary permits in accordance with local regulations.

3. Description of how the project will be monitored, and progress will be documented.

4. Detailed explanation of clearance testing procedures, protocols, and any guarantees associated with the work.

5. Advice on how to monitor and maintain the environment post-remediation to ensure long-term air quality and system efficiency.

With so many moving parts, this process can be complex, but the SOW serves as the foundation to keep the project on track. It becomes the central document that guides the team from the initial assessment to the successful completion of the work. It ensures that the project runs smoothly and helps avoid miscommunication, unexpected issues, or delays.

The scope of work is the foundation to ensure that the HVAC system and indoor environment are properly remediated and restored to a healthy state. Proper assessment and a well-drafted SOW provide the framework for achieving a verified clean system and environment. With the SOW in place, the next step is to hire a qualified contractor who can execute the plan and bring the project to completion. This document ensures that everyone involved understands the work that needs to be done and how it will be accomplished, leading to a successful project with a clear path from start to finish.

Chapter 9

Finding a Qualified and Experienced Contractor for the Job

At this stage, you may feel overwhelmed by the realization that your home, a place meant to be a sanctuary for you and your family, may be contributing to health issues. In other words, your 'home sweet home', isn't so sweet. This can be incredibly stressful. However, with the help of knowledgeable and experienced professionals guiding you through the project, there is a clear path toward resolving the issues at hand, and a resolution is within reach.

When searching for a contractor, focus on the types of projects they've successfully completed. If a contractor comes recommended, there's often a good reason. The only way to ensure consistently successful projects year after year is through a combination of continued education and training, maintaining a high standard of workmanship, daily quality control, and, most importantly, verifiable results.

This type of work is complex, much like the precision required in surgery; if it isn't done right, the consequences can be serious, with lingering concerns that could affect your health and home. In most cases, simply cleaning, remediating, or replacing ductwork or an HVAC system won't address the root issues that led to its poor condition. One of my favorite quotes summarizes this point well:

"The bitterness of poor quality remains long after the sweetness of low price is forgotten."

— Benjamin Franklin

To complete these types of projects successfully, you may need various contractors and specialists, including:

HVAC State Licensed Contractor / Certified Ventilation Inspector

Air Systems Cleaning Specialist / Ventilation Systems Mold Remediator

Certified Microbial Consultant

Certified Indoor Environmentalist / Indoor Environmental Professional

Certified and State Licensed Mold Remediator

Energy Calculations Company

Drywall Contractor

Insulation Contractor

Electrical Contractor

Roofing Contractor

Building Engineer

General Contractor

Let's explore the roles these professionals play in ensuring a thorough and effective project:

HVAC State Licensed Contractor / Certified Ventilation Inspector

This professional will assess both the mechanical functionality and hygiene of your HVAC system. They will evaluate any areas contributing to elevated humidity, condensation, pressurization, or ventilation issues. The inspection may include other ventilation systems like dryer and bathroom exhausts to ensure they are functioning properly. They will also assess whether the building structure is negatively impacting the HVAC system's operation. Based on this inspection, a detailed Scope of Work (SOW) will be created, outlining the necessary tasks, how they will be performed, and the expected results. A licensed AC contractor will be able to pull the necessary permits, as required by the state, for the replacement and installation of AC equipment, dehumidifiers, and ductwork.

Air Systems Cleaning Specialist / Ventilation Systems Mold Remediator

This AC specialist handles the actual cleaning, remediation, and/or replacement of the HVAC system, as per the scope of work. Once the project begins, containment strategies are implemented. At a minimum, Level 1 containment is set up, and the HVAC system is shut off for cleaning and repairs. Once the work is complete, the system will be sealed until clearance testing verifies that the work has been completed successfully. In cases where the contaminated system is entirely removed, the new system may not be installed until all clearance testing is completed and the results are a pass.

Certified Microbial Consultant

A microbial consultant specializes in investigating microbial issues, performing mold inspections, testing, and bioaerosol sampling. They can interpret lab results, create protocols for remediation, and conduct post-remediation testing to verify that the project was successful. Certification through organizations like ACAC is crucial in ensuring the consultant's credibility.

Certified Indoor Environmentalist

This expert assesses indoor air quality and investigates problems like mold, volatile organic compounds (VOCs), allergens, dampness, poor ventilation, and sick building syndrome. They play a key role in verifying project success through post-remediation testing.

Indoor Environmental Professional

The IEP evaluates the entire building, conducting environmental testing to pinpoint issues outside of the HVAC system. This professional provides a detailed report outlining the necessary protocols to address these concerns. Post-remediation, they return to perform clearance testing, ensuring that the environment is free of contaminants.

Certified and State Licensed Mold Remediator

The mold remediator handles the remediation of the indoor environment based on protocols established by the environmental assessor. They use containment measures, dehumidifiers and air-scrubbing equipment to manage the environment throughout the project. These projects often require collaboration between mold remediators and HVAC contractors to achieve a timely, effective result.

Energy Calculations Company

This company provides critical calculations, such as Manual J for duct sizing and configuration, and load calculations to ensure the HVAC system is accurately sized for the space. Factors like windows, square footage, ceiling height, type of insulation and R-value, roofing, and sunlight are all considered to optimize the system's performance. They can also conduct blower door tests to identify possible air leaks in the building.

Drywall Contractor

In some cases, drywall will need to be removed to access the HVAC system for repairs or replacements. In these cases, once the HVAC work passes inspection, required to close out a permit, the drywall contractor can repair and close any openings. Any drywall removed during the overall project remediation is also reinstalled at this stage.

Insulation Contractor

If attic insulation is contaminated, or if the building requires new insulation to meet code, an insulation contractor may be brought in to remove the old insulation and reinstall the correct R-value insulation.

Electrical Contractor

Electricians may be needed to install outlets for dehumidifiers, condensate pumps, and other indoor air quality equipment. In older homes, they might also need to upgrade wiring or the electrical panel to accommodate new HVAC equipment.

Roofing Contractor

If the HVAC issues stem from a roof leak or poor attic ventilation, a roofing contractor may be required to fix the roof or install features like ridge vents or solar attic fans. They can also ensure that dryer and bathroom exhaust hoods are properly sealed to prevent leaks.

Building Engineer

For more complex structural issues that affect the HVAC system and building, a building engineer may be necessary to assess and address any design flaws that are causing problems.

General Contractor

In extreme cases where kitchens, bathrooms, or entire homes need to be rebuilt after remediation, a general contractor will oversee the reconstruction process.

Client's Question: "Now that I have my inspection reports and recommendations, in what order should the work be performed?"

Having a contractor with a proven track record is invaluable in determining the correct order of operations. Contractors will review each other's scope of work and create a plan for how the project will proceed. While the order of tasks may vary depending on the specifics of the project, here is a general overview of what typically happens:

- *Day One:* The HVAC remediation company will start by setting up containment per the scope of work. Level 1 containment is the minimum level of containment for all HVAC system cleaning projects, according to NADCA.

- *Negative pressure* – The HVAC system or area of the system being cleaned should be under negative pressure to prevent particulate material from leaving the system and entering the indoor environment.

- *Protective coverings* – Clean, protective coverings should be used to protect equipment, furniture, and flooring.

- *Cleaning equipment and tools* – All equipment and tools should be properly cleaned and maintained.

- *Cross-contamination control* – Engineering controls should be implemented to prevent contaminant discharge from the HVAC system, which can result in cross-contamination of occupied spaces.

- *Backup equipment* – To prevent possible cross-contamination from negative pressure failure due to equipment malfunction or electrical power interruption, backup equipment and dedicated power should be onsite.

Once the specified work has been completed, the air conditioning system will be clearance tested or sealed until clearance testing is performed. If this work is being performed as part of an overall home mold remediation project, the mold remediator will set up containment and strategically place air scrubbers and dehumidifiers to control the environment. These two companies will discuss their scope of work and determine how to best achieve the expected end results.

- Mold Remediation Work: The mold remediation company will remove contaminated materials and perform a final wipe-down of the environment in preparation for their clearance test.

- Verification: Once the environmental assessor confirms the area is free from mold, through visual observation and testing, the HVAC system can be turned back on to control the indoor environment, containment is taken down, and the remediator's equipment is removed.

- Final Mechanical Inspection: Any permits pulled for mechanical replacement or installation will require a final inspection to close them out.

- Drywall Repair/Putt Back: At this point, any drywall repair or other necessary reconstruction work can begin.

The final and most crucial step is clearance testing. This verifies that all work was completed according to the initial protocols and that the system and environment are now clean and safe. Nothing should be turned on or rebuilt until this clearance step is completed. Cross-contamination can occur if containment is removed, or the HVAC system is restarted prematurely.

In summary, finding the right contractors and following a carefully outlined process is critical to ensuring the success of your project. Whether containment, remediation, or clearance testing verification, every step must be followed meticulously to achieve a healthy indoor environment and a fully functional, contamination-free HVAC system.

Chapter 10

Clearance Testing = Verified Results

Post-remediation verification, usually referred to as clearance testing, is an inspection conducted after a mold project to verify that the work performed followed all necessary protocols and that the remediated area is contaminant-free. It provides a measure of assurance that the system has been remediated to a Condition 1 or better. This should always be performed by a qualified independent professional who has specific experience in designing mold sampling protocols, sampling methods, and interpreting results, according to the EPA. Professional credentials can include a Certified Microbial Consultant (CMC), a Certified Indoor Environmentalist (CIE), or an Indoor Environmental Professional (IEP). The IICRC S520 defines an IEP as an individual who is qualified by knowledge, skill, education, training, certification, or experience to perform an assessment of the fungal ecology of structures, systems, or contents at the job site. Most states require this final verification in some form for mold remediation projects.

Currently, there aren't any requirements for clearance testing HVAC systems as it pertains to HVAC mold remediation. In the NADCA ACR 2021 Standard, there is a cleanliness verification to determine the presence of particulate. However, if there is the presence of microbial contamination in the ductwork and if it can't be cleaned to an acceptable level, it should be recommended to replace it.

Today, most people who are seeking assistance with their HVAC system and its effect on indoor air quality is health related. There are a few people who just want the ductwork cleaned and sanitized, and there are plenty of blow and go companies out there that can be hired. But don't take someone's word for it, that the work performed, achieved the results claimed. In my opinion, if the work is done right, there shouldn't be a problem having a mold or environmental assessor verify through third party visual confirmation or testing that the system has been successfully cleaned and/or remediated.

Offering a third-party clearance testing guarantee on projects, to ensure cleaning and remediation work has been done correctly and the HVAC equipment verified to be free and clear of any mold contamination shows that a company stands behind what they do and will verifiably achieve the results that the client was told they could expect. When all the work is complete, the final clearance testing will be performed. This clearance testing is specific to the HVAC system. The air conditioning system can't be turned back on until this test is completed because if there is still mold, it can cross-contaminate areas that are clean. If any part of the system fails, that area gets recleaned and retested. This clearance will be confirmed by the assessor performing the testing, and the job will either be cleared for operation or instructions provided for additional work that may need to be performed.

Clearance testing can include one or any combination of the following, as determined necessary by the environmental assessor performing the tests and approved by the client.

Visual and Olfactory Assessment – This is the most basic of inspections and is conducted to see and smell if the system has been cleaned or remediated to an acceptable level.

Air Sampling – This test usually involves an air pump and a collection cartridge. Mold spores, pollen, skin cells, insect parts, and fibers are often collected during this process and are used to analyze airborne particles.

Surface Sampling – This test can help identify suspect materials as mold and determine the type of mold present and at what concentration level relative to the control. This usually involves swabbing a surface suspected of contamination but can also include bulk sampling or even using tape lifts.

Wall Cavity Sampling – Using the same equipment as air sampling, this method involves pulling air from within a wall or ceiling cavity so the air can be tested for mold.

ERMI – Environmental Relative Moldiness Index uses dust samples to determine the presence of mold in an area. It uses DNA-based methods to determine the mold type.

Petri Dish Test – Often found in home improvement stores and online do-it-yourself stores, these dishes are used to observe mold growth. These aren't to see if you have mold in the environment because if you lay out a petri dish, mold will grow on it.

Be careful of companies who clearance test or sample their own work and then send that sample to a lab, claiming that the third party is the lab and that it's the lab that will be providing the results of the testing. In this case, the company that did the work is still clearance testing their own work, and that isn't ethical. An unassociated company with the project, which didn't do any of the work, is required to verify that the work was done correctly. Also be cautious of clearance testing that involves only air sampling. I have seen air quality tests that showed the air quality in the home was good; however, upon inspecting the ductwork, we saw heavy microbial contamination. How is this possible?

Sometimes a heavy fogging treatment is done within the environment. Air samples taken shortly after that treatment won't indicate accurately what is still contaminated in the HVAC system. In other cases, in an environment where the humidity is at an unacceptable level, 60% and above, common molds found in ductwork may not become airborne because they are adhered to the duct surface.

If the humidity is maintained at this level, the mold will continue to proliferate, and the environment will only get worse. One might think the solution is to dehumidify the air. Although the air needs to be dehumidified, in this case, dehumidifying the air into an acceptable range could allow the mold adhered to the surface of the duct to dry enough, and could be released into the air stream. As you can see, although air sampling is important, it is only part of an overall testing plan and shouldn't be used alone to determine HVAC mold remediation protocols or to verify the success of an HVAC cleaning or remediation project.

In conclusion, it is important to have a qualified person or company who understands all the different means of verifying that environments are clean and safe for occupancy. As it pertains to the HVAC system, several tests are performed to determine whether a system is clean. This final verification should be listed in the scope of work; what is an acceptable level of cleanliness, what test will be performed, the timeframe to have remediated areas tested, and who should be responsible for performing these tests.

Chapter 11

Equipment to Help Maintain a Clean HVAC System and Indoor Environment

It's crucial to have a thorough investigation by an Indoor Air Quality professional to identify the necessary remediation steps and determine the best combination of equipment to achieve optimal air quality for each unique environment. Even the best devices will fall short of expectations if they're not properly implemented and monitored. Every piece of equipment listed here works effectively, but without the right approach, the money spent won't yield the results you're hoping for. Here's a list of equipment used in various combinations that can significantly improve and maintain better indoor air quality:

- Central Heating and Air Conditioning System

- AC Filtration

- UVGI (Ultraviolet Germicidal Irradiation) Light Disinfection for AC Cooling Coil

- Whole-Home Induct Air Purification Systems

- Stand-Alone Air Purifier

- Whole-Home Dehumidifier or Stand-Alone Dehumidifier

- Ventilator

Central Heating and Air Conditioning System

At the heart of your indoor climate control, your air conditioning system must be correctly sized based on accurate heat load calculations. These calculations consider factors such as the size of the house, ceiling height, type and R-value of insulation, window types, and more. I've encountered numerous cases where air conditioners were oversized for the space, leading to high humidity and mold problems due to a phenomenon called short cycling.

Short cycling occurs when an oversized air conditioner cools the air too quickly, reaching the set temperature before enough moisture is removed. The system shuts off, and the humidity begins to rise again, often exceeding 60%, creating an ideal environment for mold growth.

On the other hand, an undersized unit won't remove enough moisture either. It will run constantly, leading to high energy bills, but without adequately reducing humidity because it can't handle the heat load. As you can see, both oversized and undersized systems can cause elevated humidity, which often leads to mold. When the air conditioner is properly sized, installed, and functioning correctly, it cools the air and should remove enough moisture to keep it maintained in the acceptable range.

AC Filtration

If you've ever looked into a beam of light shining through a room, you've probably noticed all the tiny particles floating in the air. Every indoor environment has a "particle load," which refers to the number of particles suspended in the air at different sizes. These particles can include dust, mold spores, pollen, pet dander, smoke, bacteria, and even gases like formaldehyde. Many of these particles are so light that they never settle from the air by gravity alone, making it easy for them to be inhaled into the lungs, where they can cause problems for sensitive individuals.

While air filters can remove particles from the air, the primary purpose of the air filter in your air conditioning system is to keep dirt from getting into the air handler. From the HVAC perspective, less filtration is usually better for system performance because it has less effect on airflow resistance. The goal in using the air condition system, to improve air quality, must strike a balance between adequate filtration (particulate removal) and system efficiency.

When a new air conditioner is installed, the static pressure (resistance to airflow) is measured using a manometer. There is an acceptable static pressure range without any filtration added. If a filter with a high-pressure drop is used (for instance, high MERV-rated filters), it can increase the system's overall resistance, which strains the system. As this filter becomes impacted, this strain on the system only increases.

Client: "I was told that upgrading my filter to a high MERV-rated filter for my air conditioner will make my air quality better. Is this true?"

There's a common misconception that upgrading to a higher-rated filter for the air conditioner will drastically improve air quality. While the filter will capture particles that pass through it, only a small portion of the air in your home ever makes it through the filter when the system cycles on and off (fan in the auto position at the thermostat). The goal of filtration from an indoor air quality perspective is to use the highest efficiency filter the system can handle, paired with regular replacement. Just because the filter says it's good for 6 months, the air conditioning system might disagree.

To achieve improved air quality, aim for 3-4 Air Changes Per Hour (ACH), which means replacing the entire volume of air in a room several times per hour. Running the blower (fan on the thermostat) in the "ON" position will help with air changes, although in humid climates like Florida, this can increase the humidity inside the house by as much as 10%, necessitating the use of a dehumidifier.

The higher the MERV rating, the more restrictive the filter. Filters that remove all the stuff they claim will become impacted more quickly. After a month of air has passed through the filter, you can have odor and bacteria build up on that filter. Excessive filter loading will cause the air conditioner to work harder. The air will take the path of least resistance and go around the filter known as filter bypass. When this happens, no filtering of the air occurs, the equipment is strained and particles entering the air handler now become a food source for mold.

Using the right filter and keeping up with recommended filter maintenance is key to the air conditioning system continuing to operate as intended. This recommendation will fail if the filter doesn't get changed on schedule. The filter becomes impacted, restricting proper air flow and increasing the static pressure within the system. If the system has a variable-speed blower motor, now standard for most air conditioning systems, the motor will run faster to satisfy the air flow required by the cooling coil. This increased fan speed pulls air through the evaporator coil much faster, causing less dehumidification and cooling to occur.

Every HVAC setup is tailored to each environment, i.e., sizing the equipment, ductwork configuration, and material selection. The filter can be a great tool for better air quality when used properly. A proper assessment by a qualified HVAC contractor should be considered and, in some cases, required to install certain equipment on the system. There are many different filter manufacturers, and other configurations can work. Here are a few filter options with a maintenance schedule that I feel is simple and works great.

Upgraded filtration with maintenance schedule.

A. 1" or 2" Pleated Filter (MERV 10-12) with or without activated carbon (formaldehyde and odor reduction). Replace the filter monthly when operated 24 hours a day. Replace in half the manufacturers' recommended time under normal operation. Individual environments may need slight adjustments.

B. 4" or 5" Extended Pleated Filter (MERV 10-12) with activated carbon (formaldehyde and odor reduction). Replace the filter monthly when operated 24 hours a day. Replace in half the manufacturers' recommended time under normal operation. Individual environments may need slight adjustments.

C. *Intellipure SuperV* Ultrafine Whole House Air Cleaner, Disinfecting Filtration System (DFS) 99% efficient for particles down to 0.007 microns. The manufacturer recommends replacing the filter every 3 years under normal operation. Replace the filter every 1.5 years when operated 24 hours a day. In some environments, the filter operating 24 hours a day may need to be replaced yearly. If the system is operated with an outdoor ventilation system, the manufacturer recommends replacing the filter every 6 to 9 months. Individual environments may need slight adjustments.

More information on filtration can be found through ASHRAE, the National Air Filtration Association (NAFA), and IAQA.

Types of Filters

Filters have many different numbers to determine their effectiveness at removing particles from the air. The MERV rating, created by ASHRAE, is one of the measures used, and it stands for Minimum Efficiency Reporting Value. It determines how well a filter is at trapping particles of a specific size. The rating is based on the smallest particle the filter can trap, which is measured in microns.

Hog Hair Air Filter – These filters can be cut to the size needed and have a high dust-holding capacity. These filters are washable and usually made of natural, durable fibers. This type of filter medium is good for the air conditioning system as it's less restrictive but might not capture all the particles in the air that pass through it. They are usually MERV 5-8.

Dust Lok – This is a very good filter medium. It includes some type of anti-microbial adhesive to control microbial growth and absorb particles. This filter is also cut-to-size and is easily replaced by removing it from the filter frame and inserting a new piece. This air filter medium is usually around a MERV 9 rating.

Fiberglass Air Filter – These filters are typically used throughout the HVAC industry. They are considered very low efficiency, barely stopping anything but large particles. They have a MERV rating of 1-4, offering less than 20% efficiency.

Pleated Air Filters – These are made of materials like polyester, cotton, or paper and have a larger surface area. With a MERV rating of 5-12, they are more efficient, trapping between 20% and 35% of smaller particles.

Extended Pleated Filters – Rated between MERV 9 and 16, these filters are designed for higher efficiency. They capture between 40% and 95% of smaller particles, making them suitable for hospitals, surgery areas, and specialized environments but are usually too restrictive for residential systems at MERV ratings above 12.

HEPA Filters – These are high-efficiency filters rated MERV 17-19, capable of removing 99.97% of particles down to 0.3 microns. While highly effective, they are not designed for residential air conditioning systems due to their airflow resistance.

Activated Carbon Filters – These filters are excellent for trapping odors and gases, such as VOCs like formaldehyde. They can help reduce smells from pets, smoke, cooking, and household chemicals as well as hundreds of other chemicals from the ambient air.

Intellipure Super V – A whole-house filtration system that removes 99% of particles down to 0.007 microns, providing superior filtration without the high-pressure drop of traditional high efficiency air filters.

Particle Size	Particle
1 to 40 microns –	Mold

2.5 to 10 microns –   Pet Dander

.5 to 100 microns –   House Dust

.3 to 3 microns –   Bacteria

.02 to .5 microns –   Viruses

.1 to 1 micron –   Tobacco Smoke (particles and gases)

5 to 200 microns –   Pollen

UVGI (Ultraviolet Germicidal Irradiation) Light Disinfection

Treating or disinfecting surfaces through exposure to UV light has been successfully used in food processing plants, kitchen sanitation, healthcare facilities, and educational facilities. UV-C is considered a very high energy and destructive type of lamp whose operating wavelength is 253.7nm. These are considered no ozone-producing lamps. Ozone can only be produced at wavelengths below 240nm (UV Resources). There are UV light systems that burn at wavelengths that produce ozone, but I highly recommend avoiding this equipment.

Ultraviolet Germicidal Irradiation, a UV-C sanitizing surface treatment light is intended for the cooling coil and drain pan inside the air handling unit. It helps prevent microbial growth on surfaces like the coil fins, where biofilm tends to accumulate. This biofilm can trap particles and harbor mold, reducing system efficiency and increasing static pressure. This equipment is preventative and does have its limitations. It isn't a one-time cure-all for the air handler. The UV light needs to be properly maintained with regular bulb replacement.

Client: "I was told by my service company that there is mold in my air handler and all I need is this UV light to get rid of the mold and improve my indoor air quality. Is this true?"

UV lights are good at preventing new growth; they cannot magically just make mold disappear. Proper cleaning of the system must be done, issues that may have caused mold contamination in the first place must be addressed, and then UV lights can be used to maintain cleanliness. UV light disinfection in the air handler is for surface treatment, not air treatment, and location is important when installing this equipment.

Whole-Home Induct Air Purification Systems

Induct air purifiers can break down pollutants into harmless byproducts like water and carbon dioxide. These systems can reduce the number of airborne particles and contaminants, such as VOCs, mold, and bacteria. However, regular monitoring is essential to ensure they work as intended. They are safe for humans and animals and are at work in many clinical, commercial, and residential buildings, including the International Space Station.

PCO, Photocatalytic Oxidation

The oxidation of pollutants is broken down into components natural to the environment, H_2O_2 (hydrogen peroxide), H_2O (water), CO_2 (carbon dioxide), O_2 (oxygen) and -HO (hydroxyl). As necessary, careful monitoring is always recommended. This technology actively disperses air-cleaning molecules and multi-cluster ions, which attach and destroy contaminants and pathogens throughout the indoor environment. This is different than the passive air treatment devices like filters which require the contaminant to be pulled through a medium for removal.

Ozone Generators

Ozone is an O3 covalent bond. It is created naturally in the environment, indirectly created by ion generator air purifiers and high intensity burning UV bulbs, but also directly by ozone generators. Ozone is considered a pollutant by the EPA and is often found in high concentrations around big cities where there is lots of pollution. When ozone encounters a pollutant, one of the atoms breaks off, leaving O2 (oxygen). The atom breaks down the pollutant into different parts of carbon dioxide, oxygen, or water, all of which are natural to the environment. Ozone in high concentrations indoors can cause headaches and, because it is a lung irritant, cause what would be comparable to a sunburn on the lung tissue.

Hydroxyl Generators

This equipment mimics ozone. These generators use UV-C to remove odors, volatile organic compounds (VOCs), virus particles, and bacteria particles from the air. These are popular remediation tools.

Ionizers

This equipment sends negative and positive ions into the environment. Some particles in the air are so light that they never fall out of the air by gravity. With ionization, these tiny particles will have a charge that will allow the particles to be attracted to one another and as they conglomerate, they become heavy enough to fall out of the air by gravity.

This technology, like the UV light, is preventative, helping maintain an already clean system. Installing this equipment into a moldy supply plenum won't provide great results, and it doesn't eliminate the mold that's there. Ask the person how they will quantify the results they are claiming. All this equipment is worth the financial expense when properly installed and the system maintained.

Stand-Alone Air Purifiers

In the pursuit of clean air, the fewer particles that are floating in the air for us to breathe, the better we should feel. Clean air is a vital part of everyday life and affects our lungs, blood circulation, heart, and overall physical health. According to the EPA, the concentration of pollutants is often two to five times higher indoors than outdoors.

These portable air purifiers are excellent for reducing the particle load in specific rooms, particularly bedrooms, where we spend many hours sleeping. Most of these purifiers use HEPA filtration and/or UV light disinfection and are very effective at removing common irritants. They complement whole-house systems by targeting specific high-use areas.

Dehumidifiers

Dehumidification is one of the single most important aspects of keeping microbial contamination from occurring within the HVAC system and the indoor environment.

Client: "What temperature should I keep in my house while I'm away for a couple of months?"

In this case, the temperature isn't the important thing. The humidity, however, very much is. The house temperature could be 100 degrees, or it could be 50 degrees, if the humidity is maintained below 50%, the environment shouldn't be conducive to mold growth. On the other hand, if the house temperature is 100 degrees or 50 degrees but the humidity remains above 60%, the environment would now be susceptible to microbial growth. According to the EPA, the indoor RH should be kept under 60%, with the ideal range being between 30-50%.

Having a whole home dehumidifier installed by a licensed HVAC contractor can greatly improve indoor air quality. This piece of equipment is dedicated to constantly removing moisture from the air, the walls, the flooring, and the furniture. Properly controlled humidity helps to fight viruses, bacteria, mold, and other airborne pollutants.

RH maintained under 48% has been noted to deter things like mites (dust mites) from living in the environment. In my opinion, the ideal range in most cases is 40% to 50% RH, depending on one's own comfort. Even though we want dehumidified air, we don't want it so dry that it becomes an irritant. In dryer climates or locations where heat is necessary most of the time, humidifiers are used to add moisture to the air.

If the indoor space isn't being cooled by a central air conditioning system or there is no place to install a whole home dehumidifier, a stand-alone dehumidifier can still be effective. Locating the stand-alone dehumidifier near an air return vent will allow the dehumidified air to be drawn into the system and dispersed throughout the house using the supply ductwork. If you must leave for an extended period of time, place the dehumidifier into the bathtub and pull the bucket out so it can run constantly while you are gone. You don't have to worry about any water leaks because the water will just go down the drain.

Ventilators

"Ventilation and Acceptable Indoor Air Quality," ASHRAE Standard 62.1 specifies minimum ventilation rates and other measures intended to provide indoor air quality that's acceptable to human occupants and that minimizes adverse health effects. Ventilation is the process of exchanging or replacing air in a space to provide better indoor air quality, which involves temperature control, oxygen replenishment, and the removal of odors, smoke, dust, airborne bacteria, carbon dioxide, and other gases.

It helps to keep the interior building air circulating and prevents stagnation of the interior air. The outdoor air should be filtered and dehumidified prior to being introduced into the HVAC system. Sometimes, there isn't a perfect solution to environmental contaminants, and the only way to improve indoor air quality is to dilute the pollutants. The saying goes, "The solution to pollution is dilution."

Most commercial buildings are required to have a certain percentage of outdoor or makeup air provided to the building to maintain a particular pressurization. This is particularly tricky when you are in a hospital setting where the maintenance closets and bathrooms need to stay under negative pressure while operating rooms remain under positive pressure and an overall neutral to slightly positive pressure on the entire building.

Bathrooms and janitorial maintenance closets are required to remain under negative pressure so the chemicals, odors, and materials inside these spaces don't enter the occupied space. The air being removed is going to be replaced in the building regardless of how it makes its way back into the building. It would be better to control the temperature, humidity, and air quality through filtration utilizing the HVAC system and other means.

During inspections of many different types of facilities, I found the outdoor air intake of the system partially or fully closed. This is done to save money by not having to condition the outside air being introduced into the system. The downside to this action is air quality problems like elevated carbon dioxide or elevated humidity due to a reduced heat load on the system. Many of the problems I would be there to help solve were created by the owners themselves unknowingly.

Elevated carbon dioxide indoors can produce a variety of health effects. These may include fatigue, headaches, dizziness, and difficulty breathing, just to name a few. Carbon dioxide is a colorless, odorless, non-flammable gas that naturally occurs in the atmosphere and through humans' exhaling. Carbon dioxide levels outside will vary depending on location, but currently, the carbon dioxide ppm is around +/-400.

The previous Harvard study also found that at 950 ppm, our cognitive performance declines by about 15%. Many metropolitan areas can be upwards of 600 to 900 ppm. ASHRAE recommends maintaining indoor CO_2 levels no greater than 700 ppm above ambient levels (assumed to range between 300 and 500 ppm). As a guideline, CO_2 inside should be maintained between 300 and 1000 ppm. At 600 ppm, there are minimal air quality complaints. 1000+ ppm could be an indicator of inadequate ventilation.

A whole home fresh air ventilator can bring outside air into the home or building. When this is incorporated into the system, I can't stress enough how important it is that the air is dehumidified prior to it entering the system. I have seen so many air handlers with excessive amounts of rust and microbial contamination that usually extend into the supply plenum and ductwork for systems that have outdoor air being introduced into the system without proper dehumidification. Ventilation is important but the air must be properly dehumidified and filtered prior to it entering the intended space, especially in humid climates.

Chapter 12

Factors That May Be Contributing to Elevated Humidity

I've already touched on several of these factors throughout this book, but let's briefly cover each one again here. Other factors may also need to be considered besides the ones mentioned here, and there is usually more than one event occurring at a time that should be addressed when attempting to diagnose or resolve these issues. Humidity is challenging, with activities from the human factor being the most challenging to understand and correct.

Air Conditioner Improperly Sized

An improperly sized air conditioner, whether too large or too small, can lead to elevated humidity levels. A unit that's too big will cool the air too quickly without enough time to remove the moisture, resulting in higher humidity. On the other hand, a unit that's too small will run constantly and still fail to properly dehumidify the space, creating the same problem. Both scenarios can cause indoor conditions that promote mold growth. When in doubt, a heat load calculation based on the current conditions of the house or building is well worth the investment.

Air Handler Cabinet Not Properly Sealed

Air handler cabinets are typically under negative pressure because the blower wheel pulls air through the cooling coil rather than pushing it. Any gaps or unsealed entry points on the cabinet, such as around the panel doors or where wires enter, become potential areas for unconditioned, humid air to enter the system. This unconditioned air can elevate the humidity inside the air handler and affect overall system performance, allowing moisture to build up and mold to thrive. Even positive pressure cabinets can experience leakage and should be sealed.

Old or Leaky Ductwork

Leaky ductwork can disrupt the pressurization of both the attic and the indoor environment. When ductwork isn't sealed properly, it allows humid air to enter the system and indoor environment, creating conditions for elevated moisture levels inside the home. Pressurization problems from leaking ducts can also cause unbalanced airflow, leading to excessive humidity in certain rooms or areas.

Clogged Dryer Vent

The dryer exhaust system typically uses a 4-inch round duct to vent the hot, humid air outside. However, if the vent becomes clogged, this moisture-laden air can be forced back into the house through the hose connections at the back of the dryer. Not only can this increase indoor humidity, but it can also cause the dryer to overheat and eventually burn out, an expensive replacement. Plus, clogged dryer vents are a significant fire hazard, with approximately 15,000 dryer vent fires reported annually in the U.S. Dryer manufacturers recommend cleaning the dryer exhaust system at least once a year or more frequently if necessary.

Dirty Bathroom Fans and Exhaust Ducts

Bathroom fans are designed to remove humid air generated from activities like showering. If the fan is dirty or the exhaust duct is blocked, that humid air remains trapped inside the bathroom. This can increase the overall humidity throughout the house and lead to moisture-related problems, particularly in the bathroom, where damp surfaces create an environment ripe for mold growth.

Outdoor Air Intake Not Properly Dehumidified

When outdoor air is brought into a home or building through an intake vent or ventilation system, it should be dehumidified before entering the HVAC system. The air conditioner alone cannot effectively cycle out this excess moisture. Without proper dehumidification, components inside the air handler, such as the cooling coil and drain pan, can become rusted or corroded, making the system harder to clean and maintain.

Attic Access Inside the House and Not Properly Sealed or Insulated

Attic access panels located inside the house should be properly sealed to prevent unconditioned air from being drawn into the home. Without proper sealing, humid attic air can seep in, raising the indoor humidity. Insulation should also be placed on top of these panels to minimize heat transfer and prevent heat loss, further reducing strain on the air conditioning system.

Attic Access Near the Air Return Intake

Attic access panels located near return air intakes are particularly vulnerable to drawing in humid attic air. When the return air pulls in this unconditioned air, it can increase indoor humidity levels and strain the air conditioning system.

Attics with Spray Foam Insulation

Spray foam insulation is a clean, effective insulation material, but it can cause issues with condensation in attics, especially in climates with chronic humidity. This moisture buildup can lead to microbial growth on the roof rafters, creating a musty odor. Sometimes, the condensation can cause water staining on the ceiling. In these situations, a dedicated dehumidifier is often necessary to control humidity levels within the attic space and prevent moisture problems.

Gas Appliance Vent Stack

Gas appliances like furnaces, water heaters, and dryers require a vent stack to allow gas and fumes to escape. This vent usually opens into the attic or outside the building. While this is a necessary safety feature, it can also provide a pathway for humid air to enter the home. Rooms with gas appliances, especially if the air return is right outside this room, should consider keeping the door closed to reduce the amount of humid air drawn into the indoor environment.

Lack of/or Poor Attic Ventilation

Inadequate ventilation in the attic can cause ductwork to sweat. Condensation can form on the outside of the ducts, and in some cases, it can accumulate between the polymeric film and the insulation in flex ductwork. Proper airflow through the attic is essential to reduce moisture buildup and maintain optimal system performance.

Lack of/or Missing Insulation Throughout the Structure

Insufficient or missing insulation can lead to heat loss, forcing the air conditioner to work harder to maintain the desired temperature. This increased workload can cause issues like sweating vent covers and moisture buildup around them, resulting in stained ceilings. Ensuring that insulation meets the proper R-value for your home's climate and construction is critical to reducing energy consumption and controlling indoor humidity levels.

Room Pressurization Issues

Room pressurization is a vital factor when it comes to diagnosing building problems. If a room or area of the house is not properly pressurized, it can lead to airflow imbalances that allow unconditioned, humid air to enter the indoor space. This not only raises humidity but can also impact the efficiency of the HVAC system. Understanding pressurization issues is crucial when identifying and resolving problems that affect indoor air quality.

Addressing elevated humidity involves a multi-faceted approach, considering factors like HVAC system performance, ductwork integrity, and insulation quality. By understanding the underlying causes of humidity issues, you can take the necessary steps to reduce moisture levels and maintain a healthy, comfortable indoor environment.

Chapter 13

Monitoring and Maintaining a Safe Environment

Once all remediation work is complete and the environment has been verified as microbial-free or within an acceptable normal ecological range, the next step is monitoring and maintaining that clean environment. It's important to remember that there is no permanent "one-time cure" for microbial contamination. Continued vigilance is key. Monitoring and maintenance will give you the best chance to provide clean air for your home or building consistently. By using a multi-pollutant air quality device, you can monitor real-time data about indoor air pollution, including particulate matter, humidity, carbon dioxide, volatile organic compounds (VOCs), and more. Actively measuring these factors allows you to manage your environment effectively. Without this information, you won't know when or where issues might arise.

This data-driven approach emphasizes verifiable results by confirming the health of your environment through verification and testing. While there isn't an exhaustive list of standards for acceptable levels of indoor pollutants, there are guidelines from organizations such as the CDC, ASHRAE, and OSHA that provide recommendations for improving and maintaining clean air indoors.

There are many types of indoor air quality monitors. Depending on the information required, it can be attained with single-pollutant sensors and multi-pollutant sensors.

- Single-pollutant sensors measure one specific air quality parameter, such as humidity, particle load, or carbon dioxide. These can be useful if you're dealing with a particular issue in your environment. For example, most people can check the temperature from a thermostat, and some thermostats also display humidity levels. A small, stand-alone temperature and humidistat device can be moved between rooms to identify potential imbalances.

- Multi-pollutant sensors, on the other hand, continuously monitor several parameters at once, such as humidity, carbon dioxide, particle load, temperature, formaldehyde, and VOCs. These provide a more comprehensive picture of your indoor environment, helping you address potential problems before they become serious. The following are only guidelines, and individual requirements will vary.

Key Parameters to Monitor for Indoor Air Quality

Particulate Matter (PM)

- PM 2.5: These are particles with a diameter of 2.5 micrometers or smaller. They should be maintained at levels between 0-12 ug/m3.

- PM 10: These particles have a diameter of 10 micrometers and should be kept between 0-54 ug/m3.

You can use a laser particle counter air quality monitor to measure the concentration of these particles in the air. Particulate control is what most people do on a daily basis with the use of filters for air conditioners and stand-alone HEPA air purifiers.

Dehumidification

Monitoring humidity is crucial for maintaining a mold-free environment. A humidistat or hygrometer can be used to measure relative humidity. Keeping indoor humidity levels between 40-50% is ideal, as higher levels above 60% can lead to mold growth. The use of a hygrometer or humidistat will be helpful.

Heating and Cooling

The temperature in the home should be regularly checked with a thermostat or thermometer to ensure the HVAC system maintains the desired climate without causing air quality issues. The system should be properly sealed at all openings and connections. The ductwork should be separately leak tested and visually assessed with a thermal imaging camera when cold air is running to check for heat loss at connection points.

Ventilation

- CO2 Levels: Carbon dioxide levels indoors should be maintained below 1000 ppm to prevent air quality issues. High levels can indicate poor ventilation.

- VOC Levels: These should ideally be kept between 0-15 ppm to minimize the risk of harmful pollutants.

- Formaldehyde: This harmful gas should be kept at levels below 0.2 ppm. Prolonged exposure to higher levels can cause health issues.

By using real-time monitoring and collecting data on your environment, you can gain valuable insights into how your indoor air quality fluctuates throughout the day or under specific conditions. For example, you might notice a spike in humidity after a shower if your bathroom exhaust fan isn't functioning correctly; or a rise in VOC levels after using certain cleaning products. This information allows you to take proactive steps to address these issues before they become major problems.

Client: "How often should my HVAC system be inspected, and what exactly should be checked?"

Routine Inspections

Routine inspections are essential for maintaining indoor air quality. At a minimum, your HVAC system should be inspected yearly, but for those with health concerns or compromised environments, inspections every six months may be necessary. These inspections ensure not only that the equipment is functioning properly but also that the entire environment is monitored and maintained effectively.

Routine maintenance

Routine maintenance goes a long way in preventing indoor air quality issues. The system should be checked for mechanical performance, proper filtration, and humidity control. Additionally, any signs of microbial growth or moisture buildup should be identified and addressed before they can lead to larger issues. Verifying that the system is free from mold, properly sealed, and that the airflow is balanced is key to preventing future contamination.

By committing to routine inspections, maintenance, and continued environmental monitoring using sensors, you can ensure that your HVAC system and indoor environment are consistently providing clean, healthy air. Minor maintenance issues, if caught early, can prevent much larger problems down the road, safeguarding both your health and your home.

Chapter 14

Final Thoughts

Achieving good indoor air quality involves far more than simply throwing a UV light into a moldy air handler, sanitizing moldy ductwork, or purchasing the priciest air filter at the local home improvement store. Having good indoor air quality doesn't have to be super costly, but if the results expected aren't achieved, that cost is even greater. It requires diligent, proactive and ongoing commitment. To maintain high-quality air, you'll need to stay on top of several moving parts: regular filter changes, UV bulb replacements, induct air purifier cartridge replacements, routine HVAC system inspections, dehumidification system upkeep, and the maintenance of stand-alone air purifying devices. The key to success lies in partnering with experienced and qualified professionals who can thoroughly evaluate your environment, address issues, and help you maintain your system and equipment for the long term.

If you were facing a serious medical issue, would you want just one doctor attempting to solve the problem, or would you prefer a team of specialists working together to get you back to health? Similarly, ensuring good indoor air quality often requires collaborative effort.

Multiple trades, contractors, and businesses must work in unison to streamline the process and achieve the results you need.

Here's a recap of the critical steps involved in creating and maintaining a successful indoor air quality project:

Properly Assess and Diagnose HVAC Deficiencies

The first step is to fully understand the current issues within your HVAC system. Identify any mechanical problems, potential contamination, or areas of inefficiency that could be contributing to poor air quality.

Inspect the Building Envelope

A thorough examination of the building's structure is essential to pinpoint other factors that may negatively affect the HVAC system and the overall indoor environment. The building's insulation, ventilation, and pressurization all play a role in maintaining air quality.

Develop a Comprehensive Plan

Once deficiencies are identified, create a detailed plan that outlines the corrective measures needed to resolve these issues. This plan should include both immediate repairs and long-term strategies for maintaining air quality.

Follow Proper Procedures and Protocols

During the remediation and repair process, it's crucial to use industry-standard procedures and protocols. This ensures the protection of both the indoor environment and the personnel performing the work. Proper containment, cleaning, and restoration methods are non-negotiable.

Third-Party Clearance Testing

After the work is complete, third-party testing is essential to verify that everything has been done correctly. This ensures that the environment has been thoroughly cleaned and that all issues have been fully addressed, providing verifiable results.

Implement Advanced Technologies

To maintain and continually improve air quality, consider integrating various technologies into your HVAC system. UVGI lights, filters, air purifiers, and dehumidifiers are all tools that, when used correctly, can help keep the environment clean.

Monitor the Environment

Regular monitoring of indoor air quality is vital. Using multi-pollutant sensors allows you to identify any emerging issues in real time so you can address them before serious problems occur. Routine testing or sampling of key areas or equipment should be considered.

Routine Maintenance

Schedule regular maintenance for all your systems and equipment to ensure they continue functioning as intended. Preventative maintenance can identify small problems before they become costly repairs or cause poor indoor air quality.

Annual Inspections

Have a State Licensed HVAC Contractor and Certified Ventilation Inspection company conduct yearly inspections and maintenance. This ensures that the system remains in optimal condition and that any necessary testing is done to verify that the air quality meets acceptable standards.

When all these elements are brought together to ensure your HVAC system is installed and maintained correctly, the benefits are undeniable. Research has shown that improving indoor air quality leads to an overall better quality of life. People experience greater productivity, sharper focus, fewer sick days, and improved well-being in environments where air quality is prioritized.

The goal isn't to live in a bubble but to stay actively engaged in understanding what's happening in your environment, why it's happening, and how to take the necessary steps to correct any imperfections. Maintaining good indoor air quality is an ongoing process, but with the right tools, professionals, and a commitment to regular monitoring and maintenance, you can create a space where you and others can breathe easier and live healthier.